'This splendid book contains practical information – clinical, psychological, social, legal, social, spiritual and ethical – combined with wisdom and background understanding so that a thoroughly holistic picture emerges. It also encourages thought about training in the complex field of end of life care for people living with dementia.'

*– Julian C. Hughes, RICE Professor of Old Age Psychiatry, University of Bristol*

'This book offers concise and practical guidance on caring for people with dementia who are reaching the end of their lives, promoting dignity and the needs of lay (family and friend) and professional carers. It offers clear learning outcomes, case studies and examples of good practice to bring this knowledge into everyday care.'

*– Dr Elizabeth Sampson, Reader, Marie Curie Palliative Care Research Department, University College London*

'The care of people with advanced dementia is an increasingly important area of end of life care. This book provides a practical and well-referenced overview of the key issues, using accessible case studies to illustrate key points. I look forward to using it in palliative care education and as an excellent source for reference.'

*– Jane Seymour, Professor of Palliative and End of Life Care, School of Nursing and Midwifery, University of Sheffield*

**University of Bradford Dementia Good Practice Guides**

Under the editorship of Professor Murna Downs, Chair in Dementia Studies at the University of Bradford, this series constitutes a set of accessible, jargon-free, evidence-based good practice guides for all those involved in the care of people with dementia and their families. The series draws together a range of evidence including the experience of people with dementia and their families, practice wisdom, and research and scholarship to promote quality of life and quality of care.

University of Bradford School of Dementia Studies offers undergraduate and post graduate degrees in dementia studies and short courses in person-centred care and Dementia Care Mapping, alongside study days in contemporary topics. Information about these can be found on www.bradford.ac.uk/health/dementia.

*other books in the series*

**Developing Excellent Care for People Living with Dementia in Care Homes**
*Caroline Baker*
ISBN 978 1 84905 467 6
eISBN 978 1 78450 053 5

**Playfulness and Dementia**
**A Practice Guide**
*John Killick*
ISBN 978 1 84905 223 8
eISBN 978 0 85700 462 8

**Risk Assessment and Management for Living Well with Dementia**
*Charlotte L. Clarke, Heather Wilkinson, John Keady and Catherine E. Gibb*
ISBN 978 1 84905 005 0
eISBN 978 0 85700 519 9

*of related interest*

**Life Story Work with People with Dementia**
**Ordinary Lives, Extraordinary People**
*Edited by Polly Kaiser and Ruth Eley*
ISBN 978 1 84905 505 5
eISBN 978 0 85700 914 2

**A Creative Toolkit for Communication in Dementia Care**
*Karrie Marshall*
ISBN 978 1 84905 694 6
eISBN 978 1 78450 206 5

# End of Life Care for People with Dementia

## A Person-Centred Approach

Laura Middleton-Green, Jane Chatterjee,
Sarah Russell and Murna Downs

Jessica Kingsley *Publishers*
London and Philadelphia

First published in 2017
by Jessica Kingsley Publishers
73 Collier Street
London N1 9BE, UK
and
400 Market Street, Suite 400
Philadelphia, PA 19106, USA

*www.jkp.com*

**Library of Congress Cataloging in Publication Data**
Names: Middleton-Green, Laura, author. | Chatterjee, Jane, author. | Downs,
    Murna, author.
Title: End of life care for people with dementia : a person-centred approach
    / Murna Downs, Laura Middleton-Green, Jane Chatterjee and Sarah Russell.
Description: London ; Philadelphia : Jessica Kingsley Publishers, 2017. |
    Includes bibliographical references and index.
Identifiers: LCCN 2016036198 | ISBN 9781849050470 (alk. paper)
Subjects: | MESH: Dementia | Aged | Terminal Care | Palliative Care |
    Patient-Centered Care | Great Britain
Classification: LCC RC521 | NLM WT 155 | DDC 616.8/3--
dc23 LC record available at https://lccn.loc.gov/2016036198

**British Library Cataloguing in Publication Data**
A CIP catalogue record for this book is available from the British Library

ISBN 978 1 84905 047 0
eISBN 978 0 85700 512 0

Printed and bound in Great Britain

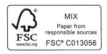

# Contents

# Introduction

> You matter because you are you, and you matter to the end of your life. We will do all we can, not only to help you die peacefully, but also to live until you die.
>
> *Dame Cicely Saunders, physician, social worker, nurse and writer, and founder of the hospice movement (1918–2005)*

## WHY IS THIS BOOK NEEDED?

The demographics of the population of the United Kingdom are changing. As medical knowledge advances, including public health screening programmes and preventive medicine, we are living longer. This is something to be celebrated, but it is not without its cost.

Humans are living for longer. Advances in medicinal diagnosis and treatment mean that life expectancy for a baby born in the UK, in 2015, is 78 for men and 82 for women (ONS 2015). The number of people being diagnosed with dementia has increased accordingly and is predicted to continue to expand. In 2013, there were 815,827 people with dementia in the UK, of whom 773,502 were aged 65 years or over; 1 in every 14 of the population aged 65 years and over will be diagnosed with dementia (Price *et al.* 2014). Fifteen per cent of all deaths between 2001 and 2009 were attributable to dementia (NEoLCP 2010); this is a significant proportion. The majority of people with dementia in the UK die in care homes where the complexity of care and challenge of fragmentation makes service provision difficult (Kupeli *et al.* 2016a).

It is impossible to imagine that traditional models of specialist palliative and hospice care will be available to all people living and dying with dementia. In fact, not all people in this situation will require specialist intervention. For many people dying with dementia, their needs are basic human requirements that can be achieved in any appropriate setting where intention, competence and confidence are supported. This book is about how to do this – it is not aimed at specialists, but at professional care providers and perhaps families who want to know how to achieve the best dying and death for the person they are caring for.

## THINKING ABOUT DEATH

In a society that prides itself on medical advancement and ever-increasing standards of living, it is unsurprising that we generally avoid thinking about death (Dying Matters 2012). For example, manifestations of a death-denying culture are seen in hospital wards where patients who are dying are moved to side rooms 'for peace and quiet', hidden from general view. Healthcare staff adopt hushed tones, and when the inevitable does occur, the finest china tea service is brought from the ward kitchen cupboard for the event of 'breaking bad news' to families and loved ones. Medical interventions are advancing at a phenomenal pace, such that it has become increasingly difficult in the Western world to die a death unencumbered from clinical interventions. So much so, there is competition for the ownership of a good death. Some campaign tirelessly through the cause of assisted suicide for the ability to choose the timing and manner of our own departing, whilst others advocate an increase in hospice and palliative care services.

But death in itself is not 'good' or 'bad' – it is merely the certain ending of the life that we have begun. Regardless of spiritual and religious beliefs pertaining to what happens next, we will all die. This does not need to be a morose topic of thought. Some faiths advocate thinking regularly about our own death and the death of our loved ones as a vehicle to reduce anxiety of the inevitable.

An ageing population has consequences for a wide range of services, and it is necessary for those services to evolve to accommodate the unique needs of the population. As people age, they are more likely to experience a range of health issues (Barnett *et al.* 2012). Barnett *et al.* (2012) further identified that as the likelihood of having a mental health disorder increased, so, too, did the chance of having a physical health problem. Whilst we do not intend to adopt a 'problem'-orientated perspective in this book, it is an important consideration that a model of single disease-specific interventions is no longer appropriate. For those people currently living with dementia in the UK (Alzheimer's Society 2012), the future is uncertain. Decisions will need to be made about where they will live, how they will be treated and who will speak on their behalf when they become unable to communicate for themselves. It is a frightening prospect.

Dementia is not a single illness. In the UK, the Alzheimer's Society describes dementia as an umbrella term for a set of symptoms that may include memory loss and difficulties with thinking, problem-solving or language. There are many different types of dementia, and neither are people all affected in the same way. People dying with dementia may exhibit a range of complex needs contingent on their individual constitution, social and demographic factors, the nature of their illness and the existence of comorbidities. These needs will inevitably change over the course of the illness, as Figure 1.1 illustrates.

The fact that dementia is a progressive, incurable life-limiting illness is not always raised. This is curious, as the typical illness trajectories of steady progression with a clear terminal phase (e.g. cancer), gradual decline with acute episodes (e.g. organ failure) and prolonged gradual decline (e.g. dementia and frail elderly) has been well described in the literature since Lynn and Adamson's (2003) seminal work about living well at the end of life. Perhaps because of dementia's prolonged prognosis, discussions about the end of life (however defined) are seldom initiated by health professionals early on. A healthcare model focused on cure means that many well-meaning professionals may not wish to draw attention to this aspect of the illness, concentrating instead on opportunities for treatment and care.

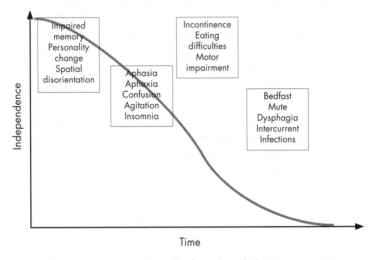

Figure 1.1 The changing needs of people with dementia over time
*Source: Adapted from Volicer and Hurley (2004)*

The fact remains that everyone will die. Some will die suddenly, without an opportunity to plan or for their loved ones to prepare. Others will experience physical illnesses such as cancer or a chronic respiratory disease, which ultimately leads to the breakdown of the physical self until the body can no longer sustain life. People with dementia may also die in these ways, but many die of the complications of advanced dementia itself: acquiring multiple infections, experiencing falls, or aspirating food through a diminished ability to swallow. This book is written for these people.

The prognosis of people with advanced dementia following acute illness is known to be poor. For example, Morrison and Siu (2000) examined the six-month survival rate of patients with dementia following admission to hospital with two common acute conditions: hip fracture and pneumonia. High levels of mortality within six months of admission were identified: 53 per cent for patients with pneumonia, and 55 per cent for patients with hip fractures. Morrison and Siu's research also identified an additional worrying trend – there was no written evidence relating to goals of care, such as decisions to withhold or withdraw life-prolonging treatments such as antibiotics. Decisions relating to cardiopulmonary resuscitation were invariably made when the patients were comatose or hypotensive and approaching death in acute hospital settings.

Whilst hospice and palliative care is a flourishing multidisciplinary specialty, there is robust evidence that care provision has failed to meet the complex needs affecting the growing proportion of people living with dementia (Ballard 2010).

The model of palliative care has evolved through experiences with people with cancer. For these, prognosis is comparatively predictable, symptom control is a frequent issue, and a plethora of evidence exists on how to manage common symptoms resulting from cancer and other physical life-limiting illnesses. There is evidence that people with dementia access less or receive substandard care at the end of life, in comparison to those who have a diagnosis of cancer (Hall *et al.* 2011; Sampson *et al.* 2006; Thompson and Heath 2013). For example, people with dementia are more likely to be admitted to hospital due to infections as well as less likely to receive pain relief (Brorson *et al.* 2014; Toot *et al.* 2013).

Dying with dementia has been termed 'the second death'. This hints at the depth of grief and loss that loved ones may feel when actual physical death threatens, having endured a similar range of emotions in response to the loss of familiar relationships and interactions with loved ones. Dementia is rarely recognised as a terminal illness. This may be due to difficulties prognosticating, or the high level of comorbidities experienced by people who are likely to be largely elderly (Birch and Draper 2008; Ryan *et al.* 2012). There is evidence that dementia is not well-reported in death certificates. For example, an international review of seven studies concluded that the reporting of dementia as cause of death was poorly reported, indicating that dementia prevalence is underestimated as well as misleading for population-based studies (Romero *et al.* 2014).

The variation in quality of end of life care (e.g. settings, age, diagnosis) has become a point of national debate (National Palliative and End of Life Care Partnership 2015) and seen in a number of key policy documents. A recent review in the UK of the Liverpool Care Pathway reported concerns that care of dying older people is not always what it should be (Neuberger *et al.* 2013). Furthermore, other examples such as the VOICES Survey (ONS 2016), that asks bereaved relatives about the quality of care delivered in the last three months of life for adults who died in England, report unsatisfactory findings related to dementia. The Care Quality Commission (CQC) thematic review on end of life care also reported unequal access to care (2016). Research in the United States looking at family satisfaction with end of life care of relatives with dementia in nursing homes demonstrated that overall satisfaction was significantly associated with communication of what is happening, including the dying process, and the perceived level of comfort of their loved one (Liu, Guarino and Lopez 2011).

The above mandate appears straightforward, but is deceptively difficult. It is known that health and social care professionals find end of life care in dementia challenging, and repeated research demonstrates a range of obstacles to provision of effective and compassionate end of life care. These include:

- difficulty prognosticating
- being unwilling to discuss death and dying
- insensitive communication
- overlooking health conditions and managing dementia, or vice versa
- difficulty assessing symptoms (see Chapter 2) or basic needs such as thirst

- difficulty identifying emotional, spiritual and social needs
- failure to plan in advance (advance care planning)
- difficult decisions about care.

End of life care for people with dementia is finally becoming a healthcare priority (Evans and Goodman 2009; Hennings, Froggatt and Keady 2010; Hockley *et al.* 2010). This book provides a tool for professionals and carers striving to enable people with dementia to live well until they die, to achieve the best possible death under the circumstances, and to maintain and sustain their own emotional and physical wellbeing.

Dementia services possess skills specific to the condition, and professional carers are likely to have insight into the person's family and personal history. Hospice and palliative care services will be able to provide advice and support related to having difficult conversations, demystifying death, and providing safe and effective symptom control whilst maximising quality of life. Hospices and palliative care services are also increasingly developing different types of partnerships to share and develop care together. For this reason, partnership working is of paramount importance when considering the needs of people with dementia as death approaches. Specialist palliative care services are not available to all, and do not have the capacity to see all people dying with dementia unless there are specific and complex needs. However, it is important not to disregard the role of such services in the provision of advice, information, education and support. For example, a single 'lunch-n-learn' session in a care home run by a palliative care nurse may be a highly effective way of improving the palliative care skills and knowledge of a range of carers. End of life 'packs' are one idea, where care homes and wards are provided with resource packs to facilitate the provision of palliative care. Suggestions for inclusion in such a pack might be the following:

- Information leaflet: identification of the 'actively' dying phase

- Forms for documentation of discussions with the person and family as end of life approaches

- Guidelines: management of physical symptoms, emotional and spiritual support

- Referral forms: fast track to continuing healthcare funding, out-of-hours general practitioner (GP) cover

- Comfort box/'Just in case' box/anticipatory prescribing

- Guidance: implementation of advance care planning, Lasting Power of Attorney and other person-centred care plans and end of life care tools as appropriate

- Pre- and post-bereavement support for family and carers

- Individualised plan of care

- Record of discussions and decisions regarding resuscitation (Do Not Attempt Cardiopulmonary Resuscitation, DNACPR).

This book offers an account of some of the challenges inherent in providing effective and compassionate end of life care to people dying with dementia. Each chapter uses current theory and evidence to develop ideas, including real-life case studies to illustrate key points. Each chapter ends with 'Key points', a consideration of dilemmas of care relating to the topic of that chapter – exploring through the use of ethical theory how difficult decisions can be made in a way that maintains personhood, safety and dignity.

Chapter 1 considers the notion of dying with/from dementia. It explores the impact of transitions in dementia and varied definitions associated with this topic, and considers some of the unique challenges posed when a person moves from living with dementia to dying with dementia.

Chapter 2 discusses some of the challenges in maintaining dignity and physical comfort in those dying with dementia. This chapter includes consideration of other conditions that may cause distress such as arthritis, and life-limiting illnesses such as cancer. Challenges in assessing physical comfort are discussed, and the use of some validated assessment tools described.

Chapter 3 focuses on emotional and spiritual wellbeing. Through the use of case studies, examples of interventions aimed at improving psychological wellbeing are discussed. The needs of people dying with dementia in different settings are compared, examining the unique challenges presented by each of these. Creative ways in which carers can connect with people via the senses are explored.

In Chapter 4 the impact of caring for people dying with dementia is considered. Common causes of stress are discussed and possible solutions offered. The ethical and legal context of decision-making (including advance care planning) is explored.

Chapter 5 continues the theme of supporting people who are caring for those dying with dementia, this time through refocusing on those professional and lay carers who undertake this role, often with minimal or no support or training. The emphasis is twofold. First, the educational needs of care staff are discussed. Second, the psychological support of care staff is explored, looking at the impact of clinical supervision, action learning sets, reflective practice, and transformational leadership and management of care settings in which end of life care is provided.

There is a lack of robust evidence on which to base end of life care in those dying with dementia. This is, in part, due to methodological and ethical difficulties in undertaking research with this vulnerable patient population. However, it is our belief that this lack of evidence does not mean that we do not know what constitutes best practice. Throughout the book, case examples from clinical practice and international innovative service development are drawn on in order to describe the many and varied ways in which professionals working in this difficult but rewarding area of practice are able to strive to continually improve the quality of life until death for those affected by dementia.

We hope that this book provides guidance, ideas, reassurance and evidence to help people to provide the highest standards of dementia care to those who are dying with dementia, to care for and about people in a way that matters and helps them the most.

# Chapter 1

# Transitions

A transition in end of life may relate to locations, settings of care, and shifts in the nature of care or people's perceptions. (For more on transitions, see Hanratty *et al.* 2014.)

## Learning outcomes

By the end of this chapter you will be able to:

- Conceptualise dementia as an incurable life-limiting illness.
- Consider definitions of hospice, palliative, end of life and terminal care, and how they apply to a person living and dying with dementia.
- Understand the ways in which people with dementia may die and where.
- Identify key points of transition:
  - Loss of mental capacity
  - Loss of ability to eat
  - Loss of ability to mobilise
  - Last year of life
  - Terminal phase of illness.
- Consider ways in which death and dying can be planned for in advance.
- Identify interventions that can enhance planning for a good death.
- Understand a range of dilemmas of care that may arise at the end of life, and an ethical framework for exploring and understanding these.

The theme of transitions highlights the value in understanding the challenges in providing good end of life care to people with dementia. This chapter outlines some of the key transitions a person with dementia (and those who are important to them) may undergo as they approach the end of life.

The median age of survival for those diagnosed with dementia is around eight years (Brodaty, Seeher and Gibson 2012; Hofman *et al.* 1991). However, dementia is rarely thought of as a life-limiting illness. Indeed, it is frequently cited on death certificates as a secondary cause of death, with conditions such as aspiration pneumonia taking precedence. However, when we consider the effect of advanced dementia on control of swallowing, for example, the two cannot be considered separately. The fact is that, even in the absence of comorbidities, dementia is an incurable illness.

This is rarely discussed. Our culture is often seen as one that denies death, that celebrates the supremacy of medicine and its increasing ability to seemingly fend off death with ever more elaborate interventions. Although, of course, this is a cause for celebration, it is also a cause for concern. Healthcare professionals may be reluctant to discuss end of life issues with people at the point of receiving a diagnosis of dementia, for at this stage hope may still be high, and nobody relishes the prospect of destroying hope. In addition, people and their families receiving this diagnosis are likely to be shocked, and require sensitive, timely and appropriate information. It may be clumsy, or insensitive, to begin to ask them whether they have considered where they would like to die.

It may be that this landscape is slowly changing. Organisations such as Dying Matters, a UK national coalition, aims to change public knowledge, attitudes and behaviours around death, dying and bereavement. It offers a range of resources for supporting this in practice, including information leaflets, posters and support for events. Russell (2014a) points out other international examples of similar death literacy programmes including Respecting Choices® (United States), Ground Swell (Australia), Speak Up (Canada) and Silver Pages (Singapore).

However, there is also much confusion over the terminology used when talking about people facing death and dying. There are different definitions of palliative and hospice care across the world (Russell 2015). For example, Hui *et al.* (2012) found 16 palliative care and 13 hospice care definitions, with supportive care rarely defined. Terminology and definitions matter because clarity at an academic and policy level and shared or agreed understandings of care structures, interventions and goals help organise and evaluate policy, experience, and clinical and research practice (Gott *et al.* 2012). To allay such confusion, these terms are now described in terms of the context of this book.

## WHAT IS 'HOSPICE AND PALLIATIVE CARE'?

The roots of hospice and palliative care lie in the work undertaken by Dame Cicely Saunders in establishing St Christopher's Hospice in 1967. In its first incarnation, the hospice was a place and a service to combine spiritual, psychological and social support with the management of physical symptoms for people dying of cancer. Hospice UK (the charity representing over 200 hospices across the UK) defines hospice care as improving the lives of people who have a life-limiting or terminal illness. It helps them to live as actively as they can to the end of their lives, however long that may be. It not only takes care of people's physical needs, but also looks after their emotional, spiritual and social needs. Hospice care supports carers, family members and close friends, both during a person's illness and during bereavement. You may also hear it called palliative care.

Cicely Saunders' foundations of hospice care were compassionate clinical care, education and research (Murtagh 2013). This model has expanded significantly over subsequent decades. In the 1980s, palliative medicine was recognised as a medical specialty in its own right, and the publication of the *End of Life Care Strategy* (DH 2008a) in the UK was the first national strategy to combine cancer and non-cancer end of life care. Since then there has been a plethora of policy documents identifying the need to provide good end of life care across all settings and all diagnoses. These include the *Government Response to the Review of Choice in End of Life Care* (NHS Finance and Operations/NHS Group/NHS Clinical Services 2016), *NICE Quality Standard for End of Life Care* (2011), the *Independent Palliative Care Funding Review* (DH 2011), *One Chance to Get It Right* (Leadership Alliance for the Care of Dying People 2014), the system-wide response to the *Review of Liverpool Care Pathway for Dying Patients* (Neuberger *et al.* 2013), and the *Ambitions for Palliative and End of Life Care* (National Palliative and End of Life Care Partnership 2015).

In more recent years, hospice and palliative care as a place, intervention or approach has been offered to people affected by other conditions than cancer, in order that all people with a life-limiting illness are afforded the opportunity for a good quality of care in their death and dying.

The World Health Organization (1998) defines palliative care as:

> an approach that improves the quality of life of patients and their families facing the problem associated with life-threatening illness, through the prevention and relief of suffering by means of early identification and impeccable assessment and treatment of pain and other problems, physical, psychosocial and spiritual.

They add that palliative care also has the following attributes:

- provides relief from pain and other distressing symptoms
- affirms life and regards dying as a normal process
- intends neither to hasten nor postpone death
- integrates the psychological and spiritual aspects of patient care
- offers a support system to help patients live as actively as possible until death

- offers a support system to help the family cope during the patient's illness and in their own bereavement

- uses a team approach to address the needs of patients and their families, including bereavement counselling, if indicated

- will enhance quality of life, and may also positively influence the course of illness

- is applicable early in the course of illness, in conjunction with other therapies that are intended to prolong life, such as chemotherapy or radiation therapy, and includes those investigations needed to better understand and manage distressing clinical complications.

Traditionally, palliative care has been the domain of specialists working with people with a cancer diagnosis. However, increasing recognition of inequities in end of life care in non-malignant conditions has led to an international impetus to expand the remit of palliative care to include all those with a life-limiting condition. However, the model of palliative care in its initial incarnation is not always easily transferable to the care of patients with a prolonged and protracted disease trajectory, such as those with dementia. Furthermore, the work on disease and dying trajectories illustrated by Teno *et al.* (2001) and Murray and McLoughlin (2012) has shown the need to closely examine not only the common pattern of an illness, but also the impact on the individual and their families. It is necessary to review ways of applying the principles in creative ways to provide care to a different demographic of patient.

## WHAT IS 'END OF LIFE CARE'?

Policy and academic literature abound with a range of terms to describe the care of people with life-limiting illness. This leads to confusion for patients and professionals alike. Ambiguity with definitions can impact on care planning and delivery. For example, a new diagnosis of dementia, with a prognosis of several years, could be described as requiring a palliative approach, according to the previous definition. But if palliative care is perceived as only symptom control in the last few days of life, such discussion is likely to herald anxieties and misconceptions. There is constant redefinition about what the time span is for end of life care. In the UK, the *End of Life Care Strategy* (DH 2008a) advocates the identification of people who may be in the last 6–12 months of life, as being at the end of life, and likely to require a range of support interventions to maximise quality of life and comfort, as this is a time which may be characterised by repeated hospital admissions and a range of physical and psychosocial issues associated with transition between living and dying. The more recent independent review of the Liverpool Care Pathway (Neuberger *et al.* 2013, p.14) refines the end of life definition, adding 'at risk of dying in 6–12 months but may live for years'. In Australia a consensus statement in 2015 defined end of life as 'the period when a patient is living with, and impaired by, a fatal condition, even if the trajectory is ambiguous or unknown' (Australian Commission on Safety and Quality in Health Care 2015, p.33).

For the purposes of this book, end of life therefore refers to the period when a person with dementia is likely to die in the next 6–12 months (but may live for years).

## WHAT IS 'TERMINAL CARE'?

Terminal care is a less frequently quoted term; it has connotations of being 'the end of the road', or the point at which nothing more can be done. However, for the purposes of this book, and to maintain clarity and distinguish between terms, terminal care is used to refer to the last hours, days or possibly weeks of life. Recent literature has started to use the term 'actively dying' to define this period in a person's life – for example, 'the terminal phase of life, where death is imminent and likely to occur within hours or days, or occasionally weeks' (Australian Commission on Safety and Quality in Health Care 2015, p.32).

In order to enable a 'good' death, it is imperative that the dying process is assessed and discussed. Dying can appear similar to a range of other problems, some of which may be reversible, such as severe infection, renal failure, opioid toxicity or metabolic disorders. Accurate and timely diagnosis is essential, as is the appropriate member of the multiprofessional team to communicate this diagnosis to others, including family.

Key principles are that:

- the wishes and decisions of the person are known or anticipated

- death is recognised as imminent and unavoidable

- life-prolonging interventions are assessed and no longer appropriate

- all care interventions have comfort and care as their primary goal

- the experiences of the family at this difficult time will have a profound impact on their grieving process.

Diagnosing dying is a complex clinical decision with many of the practice tools relating to cancer (Kennedy *et al.* 2014). It must be recognised that there will always be an element of uncertainty in prognostication, and this needs to be communicated to the family and carers. Preparing family members is important (Kennedy *et al.* 2014). For example, they may have arrangements to be made or they may need support in order to sustain their emotional and physical stamina as their loved one dies – such processes can lead a professional to try to prognosticate in a well-intentioned attempt to create order and predictability at a difficult and challenging time.

One approach that may be used is to voice your sense that time may be short by suggesting to families that we 'plan for the worst but hope for the best'.

## Key concepts

*Hospice care:* A person-centred approach to care that includes the patient and those who matter to them from diagnosis through to bereavement.

*Palliative care:* Applicable from the point of diagnosis through to bereavement. Focused on quality of life and holistic care.

*End of life care:* Identification of patients who are likely to be in the last year of life in order to plan and support care.

*Terminal care (or actively dying):* Maintenance of comfort and provision of support for the patient and family in the final hours, days or possibly weeks of life.

All of these terms represent a place, approach, intervention and philosophy of care.

# HOW DO WE APPLY THESE PRINCIPLES IN DEMENTIA CARE?

As discussed above, hospice and palliative care have their origins in the field of cancer care. Cancer is a very different illness to dementia, with prognostication (although rarely entirely accurate) and illness trajectories often characterised by a recognisable progressive decline following cessation of active treatment. There are also more services that are equipped to provide the high level of physical and emotional support that patients require.

For people with dementia, there are potential scenarios that will describe, more or less, the end of life experience – for example:

- people who already have a life-limiting illness who develop dementia

- people with dementia who then develop a life-limiting illness

- people who develop dementia as a consequence of another illness, such as Parkinson's

- people who die from the physical consequences of dementia itself.

Underpinning these possible scenarios is also the possibility of multiple comorbidities such as diabetes and respiratory or cardiac disease.

For those people in the last of these categories, the illness trajectory is likely to be characterised by increasing frailty over several years, perhaps with periods of more rapid decline associated with acute events such as falls or infections. Services are ill equipped to provide intensive support over a long period of time, and very often this takes its toll on families and carers. There is evidence that people with dementia are much less likely to be referred for specialist palliative care input at the end of life (Sampson *et al.* 2006), and fewer than 3 per cent of people with dementia die in a hospice (Hughes *et al.* 2007). Pain in dementia is often under-treated (Lichtner *et al.* 2016). Terminal restlessness is also less well-managed (Wilden and Wright 2002).

The European Association of Palliative Care (EAPC) (van der Steen *et al.* 2013) recommend that adopting a palliative approach in dementia care entails the creation of a new model of palliative care which incorporates the unique features of dementia. It advocates attention to the following issues, which will appear repeatedly throughout this book in an attempt to contribute further to the development of a new model of palliative care designed around the unique needs of people with dementia:

- decision-making
- optimal treatment of symptoms and provision of comfort
- setting care goals
- advance planning
- continuity of care
- psychosocial and spiritual support

- family care and involvement
- education of the healthcare team
- societal and ethical issues
- prognostication and timely recognition of dying.

It is difficult to prognosticate in dementia, and one of the key challenges has been identifying the point at which someone living with dementia begins to die with dementia. If dementia is a life-limiting illness, then an assessment of current and future palliative care needs is appropriate from diagnosis, at least in terms of identifying preferences and wishes, and prioritising quality of life issues. The National Institute for Health and Clinical Excellence (NICE 2016) guidelines suggest that the palliative phase should begin *at the point of diagnosis of dementia*. This would ensure that the physiological, spiritual, psychological and social aspects of care would be considered, and dignity would remain a paramount concern. Given the range of services and settings involved in providing care to people with dementia from diagnosis, implementing palliative care from diagnosis requires that the whole workforce can demonstrate effective knowledge and skills in dementia and palliative care.

## END OF LIFE CARE

A key transition takes place when someone who is living with dementia begins dying from dementia. This is termed 'end of life' and is taken to mean when a person enters the last year of life. There are no reliable evidence-based tools for prognostication in dementia, and certainly not for identifying the last year of life. Recent reviews point out the need for further research for reliable prognostic indicators in dementia (Brown *et al.* 2012). One suggestion is that this is the point at which the person exhibits a loss of communication, ambulation, swallowing and continence (Olson 2003), and although clearly this does not give accurate prognostic information, it may be helpful in identifying the potential for putting plans in place and discussing with people with dementia and their families and carers.

Guidance based on a range of available evidence and expert opinion, such as the Gold Standards Framework's (GSF) prognostic indicator (Thomas 2010), is enabling practitioners to recognise the changes in a person as they enter the final stage of their lives. A study by O'Callaghan *et al.* (2014) investigating the use of the GSF surprise question looks promising (albeit not proven to be specific to dementia).

People with dementia must show all of the following characteristics:

- unable to ambulate without assistance

- unable to dress without assistance

- unable to bathe without assistance

- urinary and faecal incontinence, intermittent or constant

- no meaningful verbal communication: stereotypical phases only, or the ability to speak is limited to six or fewer intelligible words

- difficulty swallowing or eating.

In addition, patients must have had one of the following within the past 12 months:

- aspiration pneumonia

- kidney infection or other upper urinary tract infection

- septicaemia

- pressure ulcers, multiple, stage 3–4

- fever, recurrent after antibiotics

- inability to maintain sufficient fluid and calorie intake with 10 per cent weight loss in previous six months.

Interestingly, the single question 'Would you be surprised if this person died in the next year?' has been shown to have a high level of accuracy in prognostication by general practitioners (GPs), indicating the value of intuition and clinical expertise even in the absence of more objective indicators (Moss *et al.* 2010).

## ACTIVELY DYING

For the purposes of this discussion, each chapter that follows includes a consideration of the specific situation of the actively dying person, and 'terminal' is defined as the last hours, days or possibly weeks of life.

As dementia progresses, people are likely to experience increased complications associated with their condition. Infections such as pneumonia are a common feature of advancing disease (Mitchell *et al.* 2009). The physiology behind this is attributable in part to the deterioration in the T-cells of the immune system that accompanies old age, but this is compounded by additional immunological factors in some forms of dementia (Volicer and Hurley 2004). In addition, factors such as vulnerability to decubitus ulcers as a result of prolonged sitting or being bed-bound, as well as swallowing difficulties and incontinence, add up to an overall significant increase in the risk of infections.

Diagnosis of infections may be delayed when a person is unable to verbalise feeling unwell, unless care staff or family members are vigilant for non-verbal signs such as increased confusion, behavioural change or alterations in eating habits. In advanced dementia this can be challenging. Of course, infections can be treated with antibiotics. However, there invariably comes a point where either antibiotics are ineffective due to antibiotic-resistant organisms, or their effectiveness is too late or slow to prevent death. When a decision needs to be made about whether to treat or not to treat with antibiotics, a range of ethical and moral considerations present themselves. For example, treatment with intravenous antibiotics for a patient in a nursing home may mean relocating the person to an unfamiliar environment. Quality of life considerations such as these cannot be separated from the clinical likelihood of effectiveness of the intervention.

There is a widespread reluctance to acknowledge that dementia is itself a life-limiting illness (Shega *et al.* 2003). This can lead to difficulties in having conversations with people whilst they are able to express their wishes and preferences, often leaving such decisions until too late, when carers and families are placed in the unenviable position of trying to decide on the person's behalf.

In the last weeks and months of life, meaningful communication may become more restricted, and some people appear to withdraw entirely from the interpersonal realm. This impacts on the quality of care in two key ways. First, it makes the assessment of the presence of any physical needs or discomforts challenging, such as thirst or pain. Second, there may be an impact on the caregiver. Humans exist in relation to one another, and communication is defined as a process involving more than one being. Thus it is essential that we identify creative ways to connect with people dying with dementia, maintain their physical and psychological comfort, and support their carers and families.

The National Survey of Bereaved People (VOICES) (ONS 2013), commissioned by the Department of Health, asked bereaved relatives about the quality of care received by their loved ones in the three months prior to death. The findings relating to dementia are unsettling. Almost 30 per cent of relatives stated that their loved one was treated with respect none or only some of the time. Interestingly, more relatives identified low levels of respect and dignity when their loved one had a diagnosis of dementia than when another illness was identified as the cause of death. This strongly suggests an inequality in the level of respect and dignity afforded to people with dementia at the end of life. Research in the United States looking at family satisfaction with end of life care of relatives with dementia in nursing homes demonstrated that overall satisfaction was significantly associated with communication of what is happening, including the dying process, and the perceived level of comfort of their loved one (Liu *et al.* 2011).

## WHERE DO PEOPLE WITH DEMENTIA DIE?

Sixty-three per cent of the general population express a desire to die in their own homes (Lavoie, Blondeau and de Koninck 2008). However, only around 21 per cent of people do so. This number is reduced further when the primary diagnosis is dementia (Love 2007). The vast majority of people with dementia die in care homes (around 60 per cent), compared with 30 per cent in hospitals, and only around 3 per cent in inpatient hospice settings (NCPC 2009). A worrying trend towards increasing hospital deaths has been attributed to reduced availability of beds in nursing and care homes (Agüero-Torres *et al.* 1998). Often, the point of moving someone from one care setting to another heralds a transition of one sort or another. For example, a person may be admitted to hospital from their home following an acute event requiring medical treatment. Alternatively, moving to a care home may result from carer strain or social isolation. These transitions are key opportunities for identifying what needs a person may have, and of ensuring that any existing understanding of previous needs are reviewed and updated to be appropriate and applicable.

### Dying in a care home

In the UK, around 17 per cent of people aged over 65 die in nursing or residential care homes (DH 2008a). A care home offers opportunities to create a nurturing and supportive environment to help people with dementia to live their final years and months in safety and comfort. Unfortunately, we are only too aware that this is not always the case. Recent media attention and government-funded enquiries have revealed a worrying picture of underpaid, transient care staff who are ill equipped to deal with the complexities of providing high-quality end of life care, and a lack of compassion and empathy in many centres. As people with dementia approach the end of life, it becomes no less important that their personhood is maintained. Internet discussion forums abound with stories of how people's loved ones were dressed in clothes that did not belong to them, and were left in soiled bed linen or incontinence pads, even when able to be transferred on to a commode. These basic aspects of preserving dignity are crucially important throughout the dementia journey, and represent an acknowledgement and respect for the person that they have been, irrespective of how able they are now.

Common misconceptions about palliative care that have been identified in care homes include the following:

- palliative patients are nursed in bed

- palliative care means the patients have cancer

- palliative care is the same as terminal care.

It may be useful for care home staff to consider a range of issues to enable them to identify interventions to improve the quality of life for those people who are in the terminal phase of their illness (Counsel and Care 1995).

There are many comprehensive guides on dignity for all aspects of care – for example, the Independent Commission on Dignity in Care (2012) suggests a number of standards such as listening to older people and their families and advocates. What matters in such examples is the attention to detail for the care of the individual person and their family, as well as care homes being responsible for the recruitment and education of compassionate staff.

Although often not thought of primarily as delivering palliative and end of life care, care homes have a crucial role to play in end of life care in dementia. Indeed, studies have demonstrated that the average prognosis of a nursing home resident regardless of diagnosis is less than two years, with one study illustrating that, of 1763 residents participating in a study on nursing homes, half had died within 18 months of data collection (Mitchell *et al.* 2009).

## Dying in hospital

At present in the UK, most patients with dementia die in hospitals (NEoLCP 2010). The acute admission of a person with dementia to the general hospital setting increases mortality (Sampson *et al.* 2006). There is evidence that over half of patients with moderately severe dementia admitted with a hip fracture or pneumonia will die within six months (Morrison and Siu 2000). It is difficult to obtain accurate data on where people with dementia die as fewer than half of them receive a diagnosis. Sampson *et al.* (2006) reviewed the medical notes of older adults dying in hospital, and identified over 25 per cent of these had a diagnosis of dementia. People with dementia are less likely to be referred for palliative care during their admission (Connolly, Sampson and Purandare 2012), and less likely to be involved in discussions relating to end of life care than people without a dementia diagnosis. Given the high proportion of hospital deaths ending in death, it is reasonable to assume that the real figures for the proportion of hospital deaths for patients with dementia are significantly higher than statistics suggest. Another study compared the six-month mortality rate for patients with dementia admitted with pneumonia as opposed to those who were cognisant, and found mortality rates of 53 per cent for those with dementia and 13 per cent for those without (Morrison and Siu 2000).

A study by the Care Quality Commission (CQC 2013) identified that a third of people with dementia admitted to hospital did not have anything documented on their admission record to inform staff of their dementia diagnosis. There appears to be agreement that hospitals may not be the ideal place for someone with dementia to die, but reducing the levels of hospital deaths for people dying with dementia is a gargantuan challenge. Not only does it entail educating the community healthcare teams, families and carers with regards to when to admit or not admit someone dying of dementia who becomes acutely unwell, it also entails enhancing the levels of skills in generalist palliative care. For some, clearly, hospital will be an appropriate place to be – perhaps there are significant medical health problems impacting on quality of life, or they require treatment for another condition that cannot be administered in the community setting, such as palliative chemotherapy. For those patients, it is possible to create the environment and circumstances to improve the quality of death, as long as there is recognition of the importance of this by senior staff and clinicians.

## Dying in a hospice

Hospices are designed around the principles of dignified dying, and there is ample evidence that older adults and their loved ones respond positively to this (Catt *et al.* 2005). Hospices as both a place and an approach provide a variety of in and outpatient and outreach care. In the past, hospices have faced several barriers to reaching out to people with dementia. They include low levels of knowledge about dementia among some hospice staff, and in some cases weak relationships with other health professionals, such as mental health specialists (Hospice UK 2015).

In 2015, Hospice UK (the national charity for hospices across the UK) published a series of commissioned reports that made recommendations for the future of hospice care. Within these reports the needs of hospice-enabled dementia care was identified (Hospice UK 2015). That report recognised existing best practice among a small number of hospices that provide excellent support for people with dementia through a range of innovative schemes such as inpatient admissions, outpatient care, rehabilitation, collaborations with other services such as memory clinics, as well as education. However, the report calls for this to become more widespread across the country, and provides guidance for hospice staff to develop their skills and capacity around dementia care (Hospice UK 2015). There is now increasing collaborative working between hospices and other providers to design, deliver and evaluate hospice-enabled dementia care.

## Dying at home

The majority of people express a preference to die at home, but not all achieve this goal. The proportion becomes even less where there is a primary or secondary diagnosis of advanced dementia. Numerous challenges exist in this care setting. Currently in the UK there is no full provision of 24-hour care at home. Therefore people dying with dementia are reliant on family members or other carers being present for most of the time. In an increasingly mobile population this is not always possible; adult children move away from home, perhaps having family and employment of their own. The role of the health and social care professional lies in empowering carers to support this essential role, through the availability of advice, emotional support and practical assistance.

It may be helpful for relatives to have a conversation about whether they are practically and emotionally prepared for the demands of caring for a dying loved one at home. It may be helpful to consider a set of questions to ask when considering this:

- Has the person with dementia identified their preferences for end of life care that includes being at home?

- Is reliable and responsive care available?

- Will the home accommodate any equipment that may be required (such as a hospital bed, commode, hoist)?

- Are you physically able to move the person when they become unable to change their own position?

- Can you meet your other family and work responsibilities as well?

- Are you emotionally prepared to care for your relative as they are dying?

(Adapted from Cohen and Eisdorfer 2002)

A range of innovative services have been developed to support people caring for loved ones dying with dementia at home. Treloar and colleagues developed an initiative that combined physical and mental health expertise into a home support team known as 'Hope for Home' (Treloar *et al.* 2009).[1] Referrals were accepted for any patient with a Global Deterioration Score of 8 or 9 identified by a key healthcare professional as likely to be in the last year of life, who was living at home. The service was found to increase the rate of home deaths to 75 per cent, as well as demonstrating significant cost savings. Key issues highlighted included the need for appropriate equipment such as profiling beds and continence aids. Regular review of medications, including stopping unnecessary drugs and managing difficult symptoms, was a further benefit seen in this project. The rate of unplanned admissions to hospital was significantly reduced. Facilitating carers' access to benefits such as Carers Allowance was another benefit of the project.

It is important that family members who are caring for loved ones at home are aware of how to link in with services they may require, 24 hours a day. They will require information about the dying process itself, about how to carry out tasks that may be required such as continence care, and support to help them to manage the emotional and physical demands of caring. They will also require information about what to do in cases of emergency, and what process to follow after their loved one has died. Finally, they are likely to need reassurance and validation of the immense importance of their contribution to the care of their loved one.

The Social Care Institute for Excellence (SCIE) has produced some guidance for family members about what changes to expect as someone is dying (SCIE 2012), including the following:

- Getting prepared for a death.

- How can you recognise when a person is dying?

- Final signs and what to do.

---

1    More information on this initiative can be found at www.hopeforhome.org.uk

- Offer touch and human contact.
- Provide physical comfort and care.
- Recognise and meet spiritual and cultural needs.
- Support family and loved ones.
- What does best practice look like?

## DO NOT ATTEMPT CARDIOPULMONARY RESUSCITATION (DNACPR)

Discussion and decision about whether it is appropriate to perform cardiopulmonary resuscitation is a prominent decision-making issue in clinical care. In the UK, the British Medical Association (BMA), Resuscitation Council (UK) and Royal College of Nursing (RCN) have issued updated guidance regarding anticipatory decisions about whether or not to attempt resuscitation in a person when their heart stops or they stop breathing (Resuscitation Council 2016).

The revised and updated guidance is helpful especially in terms of strengthening the relationship between advance care planning and DNACPR, and in particular how to make decisions in a person's best interests for someone with impaired capacity (Resuscitation Council 2016, p.19). This is highly relevant for a person with dementia because of the need to accurately understand and assess their wishes or decisions combined with diagnosing the end of life period, as well as discussing and communicating with the person with dementia and those who matter to them (e.g. family).

## HOW CAN WE PLAN FOR DYING?

Making and documenting decisions about preferences for end of life care is challenging. These conversations are invariably difficult, for patients, families, carers and professionals alike. Decisions often need to be made at a time when family members may be experiencing anticipatory grief, anxiety and guilt. This is affirmed by the range of perspectives from family members that can be found in the wide range of dementia discussion groups and online forums.

## Advance care planning in dementia

Harrison Dening *et al.* (2016), in a recent study (using the Quality of Carer–Patient Relationship and Life Support Preferences Questionnaire tools), identify two important points about advance care planning in dementia:

- *Dementia and decision-making:* The challenge of a person with dementia being able to consider or imagine future thoughts and actions and therefore trusting loved ones to make a decision on their behalf.

- *Accuracy in predicting wishes and decisions:* Whether loved ones can accurately predict wishes and decisions.

Harrison Dening *et al.* (2016) acknowledge that whilst advance care planning is challenging for the above reasons, and that more research is needed to understand the complexity of advance care planning, it does still offer benefits such as initiating conversations.

In England and Wales, advance care planning is a voluntary process, and there is no legal requirement for an individual to carry out advance care planning. However, the evidence supports that when wishes and decisions are contemplated, discussed, documented and shared in advance, an individual is more likely to die in their preferred place of death. It may also support people and their families as they face their mortality. There are several healthcare elements to advance care planning (as an activity) that may result in an advance care plan, including one or more of the following components:

- *Advance Statement – for example, Preferred Priorities for Care, Thinking Ahead and other forms of documents:* A written or verbal expression of wishes and choices about care at the end of life. Is not legally binding, but indicates a person's wishes as well as that they have thoughts about their future death. Useful as triggers for conversations as well as advancing more legal documentation.

- *Advance Decision to Refuse Treatment (ADRT) (other international terms include Advanced Directives and Advanced Health Directives):* A written document stating in advance what healthcare interventions an individual does not want in the future. Only comes into force if people are unable to say themselves what they do not want, and is applicable to the decision being made at the time.

- *Lasting Power of Attorney (other international terms include Enduring Power of Attorney):* Formal appointment of a surrogate decision-maker who must be consulted about two types of decisions – Health and Welfare (only comes into force if people are unable to say themselves what they want at the time), and Property and Affairs (comes into force any time that the individual authorises them).

- *Do Not Attempt Cardiopulmonary Resuscitation (DNACPR):* A medical decision not to attempt resuscitation if the attempt is felt to be medically futile or not in the person's wishes, as in a documented ADRT.

- *Treatment Escalation Plan (TEP) or similar:* Documentation of discussion and decision of what to do/not do regarding future medical interventions – for example, admission to hospital.

- *Best interests/benefit to patient:* Discussion and decision process in order to make a decision in the best interests of the person.

Ideally, advance care planning will already have been considered and discussed. However, even in the absence of care planning, it is possible to make collaborative decisions in somebody's best interests if it appears that death is near. For example, are they in the most appropriate place? If in hospital and still receiving active treatment such as intravenous (IV) antibiotics, is it appropriate to consider withdrawal of treatment? What is their quality of life like? Have any previously expressed preferences been discussed or documented either by a family member or health or social care professional? There is guidance available to help support this decision-making process (see, for example, Black 2011; GMC 2010; NCPC 2011; Resuscitation Council 2016). Acknowledging the ongoing uncertainty of prognosis is vital, particularly if the person is still receiving active treatment such as antibiotics.

In reality, the time of diagnosis of dementia is rarely the time when discussions about end of life take place. Prognosis is hugely variable at this point in the journey. Advance care planning is known to reduce the likelihood of unwanted interventions or admissions later on in the illness trajectory (Baker, Leak and Ritchie 2012), but actually taking that leap of faith and broaching the subject of mortality with a person who has been newly diagnosed with a condition is another matter. They may not die of their dementia – another condition may cause a more rapid deterioration before significant loss of capacity. Or they may die of a condition complicated by their dementia. A further option is that they may die of the effects of dementia itself, on their mobility and functioning, and eventually on those very functions that sustain life: eating and breathing. What is common to all three of these options for end of life is that in all of them the person is dying 'with' dementia. As such, consideration of their needs requires a particular focus on how this will impact on their care and decisions.

## Components

### Advance Statements

One of the ways to support people with dementia and their advance care planning is to consider completing a document such as an Advance Statement. Whilst it is not a legally binding document (in England and Wales), what it does offer is evidence that a person has thought about their end of life as well as insights into what their wishes or decisions might be. Examples that have been used in dementia include the following:

- The Alzheimer's Society document entitled 'This is me',[2] which could accompany people if, for example, they need to be admitted to hospital.

- The Butterfly Scheme[3] is a further innovation that provides people with a personalised record of their wishes and preferences that alerts staff to important features of caring for that person.

- *Preferred Priorities for Care* (NHS England 2011) is intended to relate both to wishes around medical and nursing treatment, but also to express wishes relating to activities of living. For example, it may inform caregivers of whether the person likes a particular face cream to be applied, or what music they like to listen to, or other factors that could be used to improve their quality of life if they are unable to express these preferences themselves.

## Advance Decision to Refuse Treatment (ADRT)

There are a variety of international terms, documents and legal frameworks where a person can document any treatment they wish to refuse in the future (if they cannot say so themselves at the time). In England and Wales, under the Mental Capacity Act (2005), it is possible for an adult over the age of 18 to complete a document stating in advance any future specific treatments they wish to refuse. This is known as an Advance Decision to Refuse Treatment (ADRT), and it must comply with the Mental Capacity Act,[4] be valid and apply to the

---

2   See www.alzheimers.org.uk/thisisme

3   See http://butterflyscheme.org.uk

4   See www.nhs.uk/Conditions/social-care-and-support-guide/Pages/mental-capacity.aspx

situation. Examples of decisions may include a wish to not be given enteral feeding or antibiotics, or a desire not to have cardiopulmonary resuscitation.

### Lasting Power of Attorney[5]

If the person with dementia so wishes, it is possible to legally nominate somebody to speak on their behalf in relation to both financial and health issues. Internationally there are a number of legal frameworks within which attorneys operate, and it is important to understand their content and legal jurisdictions. In England and Wales there are two types – Health and Welfare (which comes into force when the individual no longer has capacity), and Property and Affairs (which can be actioned at any time that the individual requests). There is a charge for appointing an attorney, and it can take 6–8 weeks for the documents to be processed and validated through the Office of the Public Guardian, so it is worth taking this into consideration.

## WHAT TO DISCUSS IN ADVANCE CARE PLANNING?

Whatever the person wants to! However, it is useful to think about what type of conversation is happening – for example, contemplating, discussing or deciding? Then consideration needs to be given to documenting the wishes and decisions of the person and disseminating these choices to those who matter to the person as well as to health and social care professionals. There is value in regularly inquiring if wishes and choices remain the same as well as a therapeutic space in which the person can discuss their thinking and thoughts about their future dying.

Some ideas are as follows – these are taken from a range of documents and online discussion forums, and represent a synthesis of the 'important things' to think about:

---

5    For more information, see www.gov.uk/power-of-attorney/overview

What if...

- you became more ill – where do you want to be cared for?

- you become unable to safely swallow food – would you want to be fed with a tube into your stomach?

- you develop an infection – would you like to be admitted to hospital for treatment or would you prefer treatment here (home/care home)?

What do you think...

- about what we need to do if you became more unwell?

- about what your family or friends might want to know?

- about what your family or friends might think about this conversation?

What...

- else do I need to know about you?

- are you worried/not worried about?

- matters most to you now or later?

Other examples of questions include Atul Gawande's (2014) five key questions. First:

1. What is your understanding of your current health or condition?

2. If your current condition worsens, what are your goals?

3. What are your fears?

4. Are there any trade-offs you are willing to make or not?

And later:

5. What would a good day be like?

There are a variety of other conversation tools that may help such discussions – for example, the Fink Advance Care Planning cards.[6]

## Case study: Advance care planning

Jack is 85 and has lived with dementia for six years. His capacity varies on a day-to-day, hour-by-hour basis, but his daughter Mary can see that he is worried about something. Jack starts talking a lot about his wife who died ten years ago. Mary wonders if he is thinking about his own funeral. Using the Fink Advance Care Planning cards, she asks her father to pick a card. He picks one out about who he wants to speak at his funeral. He reminisces about his wife's funeral and how he looked after her. As he carries on he reveals that he is worried about what would happen if his heart stopped. He wants to die at home. Mary arranges for Jack and herself to go and see his GP so that he can discuss what matters to him when he is actively dying. The GP talks to Jack about his thoughts. She uses questions such as: 'What if your heart stopped – what would you want us to do?' She also asks Jack: 'If you had a chest infection, would you not have antibiotics and possibly die at home, or go into hospital and have antibiotics?' Together they discuss and document a DNACPR form, and decide what other treatments not to give in the future (e.g. antibiotics). Whilst the GP was talking to Jack she was assessing his mental capacity and came to the conclusion that whilst he was able to make a competent decision about DNACPR with her in that moment, he was not able to go home and complete an ADRT form because he lacked sustained concentration and recall. Mary, Jack and the GP discuss the DNACPR, and also note on his medical records his wishes about his preferred place of death.

What does this example illustrate? It reflects an approach to care where observation of a person's usual behaviour, using person-led triggers (Fink Advance Care Planning cards and relating to the person's experience), enabled conversation about what mattered most to Jack. Moreover, the GP, using clinical judgement, made a decision about the best type of advance care planning for Jack (i.e. a DNACPR decision rather than an ADRT).

---

6    See http://finkcards.com/products/advance-care-planning

## HOW CAN WE MAKE ETHICAL DECISIONS?

The care of people with dementia involves frequent dilemmas of care. These are presented throughout the book in relation to the topic of each chapter. By way of background knowledge, a brief discussion of ethical theory is necessary.

Important key principles are those of autonomy, beneficence, justice and non-maleficence (Beauchamp and Childress 2001). The table below shows an ethical decision-making grid that can be considered when thinking about the case scenarios that are discussed in each of the chapters that follow.

| | |
|---|---|
| *Autonomy* <br> The right of the person to have a say in what is happening to them | *Beneficence* <br> The imperative to act in the person's best interests |
| *Non-maleficence* <br> The imperative to do no harm | *Justice* <br> The right of the person to be treated fairly |

### Case study: An example of key principles in ethical decision-making

Daisy has Down's syndrome and developed early-onset dementia when she was 42. She has been living in a care home for the past five years. She was deteriorating rapidly, and had had several hospital admissions with chest infections over the previous months. She has now become bed-bound, doubly incontinent and completely unable to communicate verbally. She spends most of her time asleep, and even when she is awake her eyes are usually closed. Her mother and sister feel that they would like her to come home for her remaining life, and approach Social Services to discuss any care support that they may be entitled to in order to do this. Daisy's mother has severe arthritis and her sister works four days a week. The social worker feels that this move would be risky given the complexity of Daisy's needs; he is worried that there will be less availability of medical and nursing input at home compared to that in the nursing home. He feels Daisy is well supported in the nursing home and that she should remain there for terminal care. He proposes a Best Interests meeting to discuss the issues.

- *Autonomy:* What wishes, if any, has Daisy expressed prior to losing her capacity to communicate? How are her relationships with her mother and sister?

- *Beneficence:* What is the right thing to do? Will the quality of Daisy's remaining days be improved through her being in the continuous presence of her family?

- *Non-maleficence:* Will transferring Daisy home lead to a reduction in the quality of her care? Are we certain that such decisions are not being made on financial grounds alone? Are there unacceptable risks involved in this transfer? Can these be mitigated in any way?

- *Justice:* Daisy has a right to care in an appropriate setting, regardless of her diagnosis.

Ethical decision-making grids do not provide answers, but they do present a structure for consideration of the range of issues that can sometimes help families and caregivers to reach a mutually satisfactory decision.

Daisy and Jack's examples in this chapter illustrate the value of knowing the person with dementia and taking the time to discuss with them what matters most to them.

## Key points

- We have explored how living with dementia is concerned with a series of transitions and its associated implications.
- The challenge of identifying the dying phase and defining end of life, hospice and palliative care has been raised.
- The value of approaching care through the eyes and experiences of people with dementia and those who are important to them has been demonstrated.

Chapter 2

# Physical Wellbeing and Dignity

**Learning outcomes**

By the end of this chapter you will know about:

- Person-centred approaches to the holistic assessment and management of pain and distress for people with dementia.
- The difference between dementia, delirium and terminal restlessness.
- Appropriate use of antipsychotic medication to alleviate distress.
- Some reasons a person with dementia may stop eating and drinking, and how to tailor their care appropriately.
- Appropriate and effective ways of administering the essential medications for end of life care (including analgesics, antiemetics, anxiolytics, anticholinergics and antipsychotics).
- Providing 'comfort measures' at the end of life, including physical care.

People with dementia may move towards the last days or weeks of their life at any point on their dementia trajectory. They may have mild or moderate dementia, but are in the end of life phase of another comorbid condition such as heart failure or cancer, or they may have reached end-stage dementia and be dying from the complications arising from severe physical and cognitive impairments. In end-stage dementia, immobility, incontinence and swallowing difficulties give rise to repeated infections such as urinary tract infections, chest infections and pressure ulcers, while extreme frailty impedes recovery from physical illness. Pneumonia is the ultimate cause of death in up to two-thirds of people with dementia (Alzheimer's Society 2012).

Palliative care is:

> an approach that improves the quality of life of patients and their families facing the problem associated with life-threatening illness, through the prevention and relief of suffering by means of early identification and impeccable assessment and treatment of pain and other problems, physical, psychosocial and spiritual. (WHO 1998)

While it is not always possible to remove all psychological suffering, it may be therapeutic for this suffering to be expressed. This can only happen when there is effective control of physical symptoms (Stedeford 1987). This chapter provides an overview of care practices, which aims to ensure that people living and dying with and from dementia do so in dignity and comfort.

## Key concepts

*Discomfort/distress:* A condition of either physical pain or affective discomfort; physical pain is an unpleasant internal state that results from physiological stimuli, and affective discomfort is an unpleasant internal state resulting from non-physiological stimuli (Kovach *et al.* 1999).

*Total pain:* The physical, social, psychological and spiritual dimension of suffering. A person's distress is rarely the result of a single cause (Saunders 1967).

*Behaviour:* An expression of unmet need in people with dementia. Through exhibiting certain behaviours, a person with dementia may be demonstrating a need for physical comfort, stimulation or emotional belonging (Downs, Small and Froggatt 2006).

## PHYSICAL SYMPTOMS AT THE END OF LIFE

Physical symptoms in advanced dementia can range from double incontinence and multiple comorbidities such as diabetes and hypertension (Poblador-Plou *et al.* 2014) to pain and behavioural disturbances (Sampson *et al.* 2015). Other commonly reported symptoms include dyspnoea, depression, anxiety, hallucinations and delusions (Lyketsos *et al.* 2002; van der Steen 2010). The combination of behavioural and cognitive disturbances contributes to the need for the accurate assessment of physical (as well as emotional, psychological and spiritual) symptoms.

*Physical pain* is a common symptom of advanced illness and also persists in many chronic conditions associated with ageing. The prevalence of persistent pain in older adults is estimated at 25–86 per cent (DeWaters, Popovitch and Faut-Callahan 2003). It is often compounded by factors of immobility and susceptibility to infection at the end of life (Collett *et al.* 2007).

*Breathlessness* may be the result of lung or heart disease, pneumonia, anaemia or anxiety.

*Nausea and vomiting* may be caused by bowel disease, constipation, the side effects of medications, general debility or anxiety.

## PERSON-CENTRED ASSESSMENT OF SYMPTOMS

### Why is it important?

The complexity of symptom assessment in people with dementia is highlighted by reports that pain in hospitalised patients with cognitive impairment is under-reported and under-treated (Buffum *et al.* 2007; Sampson *et al.* 2015). One study showed that people with hip fracture and advanced dementia received only a third of the analgesics administered to their cognitively intact counterparts (Morrison and Siu 2000).

## Key issues

Impeccable and careful assessment is a key part of the palliative care approach including involving the person themselves as well as their family and carers. The wider multidisciplinary team across all the care settings, such as hospice, community or hospital specialists in palliative care, general practitioners (GPs) and care of the elderly teams, are also able to advise on the management of specific symptoms as well as provide a forum for joint discussion and decision-making. For example, St Giles Hospice in Staffordshire developed a joint memory clinic with a local GP (Hodges 2015), and St Cuthbert's Hospice in Durham appointed the first ever hospice Admiral nurse in 2015 (Tolman 2015). Whilst hospices and specialist palliative care services still need to develop and extend further partnership working in dementia care, these examples show promise and development.

People with dementia are likely to have short-term memory loss and communication difficulties. As a result, these specialists also need to take into account information obtained through ongoing assessment made by their family and familiar carers who tend to have an intuitive understanding of the distress behaviour, and to detect and monitor symptoms through daily contact and knowledge of the person they care for (Hendrix et al. 2003; Regnard et al. 2007).

Holistic assessment is essential, as emotional distress and physical symptoms are often interrelated. People with dementia can have poor comprehension of the current situation and can misinterpret the environment. This can, in turn, heighten fear and anxiety (Rewston and Moniz-Cook 2008), which can lead to an increase in a person's perception of physical pain (Melzack and Wall 1967) and may induce nausea and breathlessness.

Multiple methods should be used to gather information about the person from a range of sources (Hadjistavropoulos et al. 2008; Snow et al. 2004). People with dementia are likely to experience difficulties understanding, expressing and recounting their feelings. A recent systematic review reported the importance of using pain assessment tools in dementia that are able to record pain scores over time, ability to assess facial gestures, body movements and changes in behaviour, as well as appropriate regular analgesia (Husebo, Achterberg and Po 2016). As such, person-centred assessment is a bit like a jigsaw puzzle, where the greater the number of pieces of information, the clearer the overall picture.

## Case study: The importance of accurate symptom assessment

Consider the use of analgesics for managing pain. Different types of pain (tissue, bone, nerve, muscle, organ) are responsive to different types or combinations of analgesics and adjuvant medication.

Nausea and vomiting caused by reduced gut motility and constipation would require a different management plan to nausea and vomiting caused by anxiety.

## ASSESSING PAIN IN PEOPLE WITH DEMENTIA

The unique experience of dementia makes it difficult to take a standardised approach to pain assessment, and more validated measures still need to be further investigated for agreement, responsiveness and interpretability (Ellis-Smith *et al.* 2016). Pain is often under-detected and under-treated in people with dementia, and it is important to both accurately assess and implement correct pain control (Sampson *et al.* 2015). Pain assessment guidelines need to support people with different levels of cognitive impairment, and people with fluctuating levels of cognition, while taking account of psychosocial influences.

Kitwood (1990) identifies dementia as a dialectical process in which there is interplay between neurological impairment and psychosocial factors. In this respect a person's abilities to communicate can be enhanced through a supportive environment and equally be inhibited through negative attitudes. The Mental Capacity Act (2005) states that all practicable steps should be taken to support people with cognitive impairment to express their feelings. People with dementia who can communicate verbally could benefit from supportive communication techniques such as using gestures and visual aids, asking short questions, allowing a response time, addressing sensory impairments, minimising distractions and seeking confirmation about any assumptions made (SCIE 2009). As dementia progresses and a person's verbal communication skills diminish, a greater reliance is placed on observations of their behaviour to detect their distress.

It is important to ask a person about their pain in the first instance, as a person's self-report is the most reliable indicator of this subjective experience (McCaffery 1968). Some people with dementia may find it difficult to initiate conversations about their pain if they are not asked about it or they may be concerned about bothering staff or family. Everyone should routinely be asked regardless of level of cognitive impairment, as there is no identified cut-off point that determines whether or not a person is able to report the presence of pain, which at a minimum may be by deliberate demonstration such as a nod or hand squeeze. Questions about pain should include alternative words to pain as well, such as aching, hurting, sore and uncomfortable, as the word 'pain' may be reserved for more acute episodes. A person with dementia should only be asked about their present pain, and the assessment should be made during periods of activity as well as during periods of rest. This is because, in many musculoskeletal conditions, pain is encountered on movement and may be forgotten by the person when they are not active (Collett *et al.* 2007; Hadjistavropoulos, Fitzgerald and Marchildon 2010).

While a large proportion of people with dementia are able to communicate the presence of pain, observing their behaviour remains an important part of the pain assessment (Collett *et al.* 2007; Snow *et al.* 2004). They may, for example, report that they have no pain, but if their behaviour indicates they are distressed, it may prompt further questions about pain using alternative words as well as consideration of other causes of distress. Their levels of cognition can fluctuate so that while they may be able to report on their pain at one time, at other times they may not be able to. The very presence of pain can be so overwhelming at times that it hinders a person's ability to respond to pain assessment questions.

There are a variety of pain assessment guides and tools, including the Abbey Pain Scale, the Disability Distress Assessment (DisDAT) Tool and the Pain Assessment in Advanced Dementia (PAINAD) Scale. A review by Jordan *et al.* (2012) points out that PAINAD also picks up distress that is not caused by pain. DisDAT picks up a broader array of signs, which may be useful both in practice and in research. In the UK, the National Council for Palliative Care has also produced a useful guide to pain and distress called *How Would I Know? What Can I Do?* (NCPC 2012).

## Self-report pain assessment tools

Self-report pain assessment tools are used to gain an understanding of the severity, nature, quality and location of the pain along with its emotional and psychosocial impact to aid diagnosis, evaluate the effectiveness of treatments and determine appropriate interventions of a multidisciplinary team (Twycross and Wilcock 2001). To support people with dementia, they should be in a visual form, as written words and pictures can enhance comprehension of the spoken word and reduce demands on a person's language skills and memory (Bourgeois *et al.* 2001; Murphy, Gray and Cox 2007). Clear pictures and large print on unlaminated pastel card avoids reflection and glare from white paper, but allows an adequate contrast between the background and the writing and pictures to account for sensory and cognitive deficits in people with dementia (Collett *et al.* 2007; Hadjistavropoulos *et al.* 2010).

Another approach to assessing pain is using a body map, as described by Melzack (1987). This is an outline of a body, front and back. The person is asked to point to their own body or the picture of a body to show where their pain is, and this area is marked on the picture. If they identify more than one area of pain, then the different areas are numbered.

This map should be kept in front of them when an assessment is made of their pain, to help them focus on one area of pain at a time. In addition to body maps, pain intensity scales, descriptors and charts can be used to help assess pain in a person with dementia;

- *Pain intensity scales:* Numerical Rating Scale (NRS, Kremer, Atkinson and Ignelzi 1981); Verbal Rating Scale (VRS, Keele 1948); Iowa Pain Thermometer (IPT, Herr *et al.* 2007). These should be used before and after pain management interventions to determine how effective the intervention is. The person should be asked to point to the level on the scale that represents their current pain. Vertical scales are more easily understood and minimise misinterpretation in patients with visual spatial neglect (Collett *et al.* 2007; Wilson *et al.* 2008).

- *Pain descriptors (words, or words and pictures):* Pain descriptors are words used to help a person describe the nature and quality of their pain (Bennett 2001; Melzack 1987). They include words like gnawing, sickening, throbbing, cramping, shooting, sharp, heavy, burning, stabbing, pins and needles, and electric shock. The person should be asked to point to the ones that represent their pain. Their description of their pain can be summarised using the words they have chosen, and confirmation should be sought that this is correct.

- *'How do you feel?' chart:* This comprises faces and words representing different emotions. It should be used in the same way as the pain descriptors to determine how the person is currently feeling.

Preferences for different types of pain assessment tools will vary from person to person. These may depend on a person's pre-existing educational skills, personality and culture, as well as level of cognitive impairment (Curtiss 2010; DeWaters *et al.* 2003). For example, a person who is used to working with numbers may prefer a numerical rating pain scale, whereas the pain thermometer is more visual and less dependent on a person's numeric and literacy skills. It may be necessary to trial the use of different tools to find the most appropriate for that person. This should be done when their pain is least severe (DeWaters *et al.* 2003; Wilson *et al.* 2008).

For people with visual spatial neglect, it is important to ensure the tools are displayed within their field of vision. To use these tools, the person with dementia needs to recognise the words and pictures and understand the iconicity and concepts of the pictures and scales. Working with them, it is usually possible to gauge which, if any, of the tools can be used appropriately. Confirmation should be looked for if assumptions are made about what the person is saying. The information gained should be part of a multimethod approach to pain assessment.

### Case study: A lady with dementia using the visual pain assessment tools

Ruby had peripheral vascular disease and mild-to-moderate dementia. She was able to report that she had pain in both her legs. She had word-finding problems, which made it difficult for her to express how she felt. The words and pictures of pain descriptors and emotions helped her, and she seemed to appreciate that time was taken to support and listen to her. She looked through the pictures and indicated that her pain was sharp and burning and it went down each leg. This information confirmed that the treatment she was due to commence for neuropathic pain was likely to be appropriate. She pointed to the emotions of feeling anxious and feeling frustrated. Exploring these feelings further, she was able to say that she was frustrated because she was not dying quick enough. When asked if she was anxious about dying, she replied that she was not, but she was anxious that the pain would not leave her. Through this approach the conversation focused on her total pain, and enabled her to express her feelings.

## UNDERSTANDING BEHAVIOUR

When people with dementia are unable to express their feelings verbally or with the use of supportive communication techniques, it is necessary to observe their behaviour to identify whether they are distressed. As there is no specific behaviour that distinguishes pain from other causes of distress in people with severe communication difficulties, when distress is identified it is necessary to determine the cause, which may be physical pain or discomfort, or psychosocial or spiritual causes (Regnard *et al.* 2007). It is important to exclude other causes of distress before assuming that it is because of pain, particularly if opioids are being prescribed, as they can mask other symptoms, exacerbate confusion and cause constipation (NCPC 2009).

Kitwood (1990) advises that knowing about a person, including their life story, can help care staff use imagination and empathy to provide a person-centred approach to care that promotes agency. This can help care staff anticipate a person's needs and identify and respond to possible causes of distress.

The following can be used to help understand behaviour.

### 'This is me' leaflet[1]

Families are asked to fill out this leaflet to provide as much information about the person's habits, routines and life story, the activities they enjoy and the things that cause them distress. This will help care staff to understand a person's behaviour in context. It could help differentiate between pain and other causes of distress such as hunger, fatigue and anxiety. As people with dementia often try to make sense of a situation by drawing on their memory of the past, knowing something of their life story can help care staff respond appropriately to their behaviour and understand the emotion that is being displayed.

### Disability Distress Assessment (DisDAT) Tool (Regnard *et al.* 2007)

The DisDAT is a behavioural assessment tool used to detect distress in people with dementia and severe communication difficulties. It works on the premise that distress is identified as a change from the person's normal behaviour, and in some cases

---

1    See www.alzheimers.org.uk/thisisme

it is demonstrated merely as an absence of content behaviour. The DisDAT documents a person's content and distressed behaviour, aiding the detection of distress behaviours unique to the individual. This avoids a person's distress being overlooked (Regnard *et al.* 2007). It is important to understand that what may be content behaviour for one person, such as sitting still and being quiet, could be distressed behaviour for another if, for example, they were normally active and vocal.

The DisDAT provides categories and words to help family carers and care staff record their observations of the person's behaviour. Once a person's distressed behaviour is understood, it becomes easier for care staff to pick up on episodes of distress. It offers a way for families and familiar carers to provide healthcare professionals with an ongoing record of evidence to aid assessment. The DisDAT also offers a clinical decision checklist to help determine the cause of distress (Regnard *et al.* 2007).

### DisDAT Clinical Decision Checklist

Is the new sign or behaviour:

- Repeated rapidly? Consider:
  ○ Pleuritic pain (in time with breathing).
  ○ Colic (comes and goes every few minutes).
  ○ Repetitive movement due to boredom or fear.
- Associated with breathing? Consider:
  ○ Infection, chronic obstructive pulmonary disease (COPD), pleural effusion, tumour.
- Worsened or precipitated by movement? Consider:
  ○ Movement-related pains.
- Related to eating? Consider:
  ○ Food refusal through illness, fear or depression.
  ○ Food refusal because of swallowing problems.
  ○ Upper gastrointestinal (GI) problems (oral hygiene, peptic ulcer, dyspepsia) or abdominal problems.

- Related to a specific situation? Consider:
  ◦ Frightening or painful situations.
- Associated with vomiting? Consider:
  ◦ Causes of nausea and vomiting.
- Associated with elimination (urine or faecal)? Consider:
  ◦ Urinary problems (infection, retention).
  ◦ GI problems (diarrhoea, constipation).
- Present in a normally comfortable position or situation? Consider:
  ◦ Pains at rest, infection, nausea, anxiety, depression, anger.

## Case study 1: Using the DisDAT to understand fear

Gladys had end-stage dementia and was cared for in bed. Every time care staff went to move her position, her body and limbs would become rigid, and her breathing would become faster and shallow. Her eyes would be wide open and not blinking. She had a transdermal analgesic patch giving her continuous pain relief for arthritis. At first the care staff thought that this must not be strong enough and she was experiencing pain when they were moving her.

The care staff used the DisDAT to record her behaviour over a period of time, and they discovered that when she was content her body relaxed, she would make eye contact and smile, and she would move her limbs freely. This was especially the case when her daughter visited and she would reach out to embrace her.

The care staff asked her daughter to stay while they attended to her in bed, and while she was embracing her daughter she was helped to roll from side to side in bed in order to change the bed sheet. During this time she remained relaxed and content.

It was concluded that her distressed behaviour was a result of fear when being moved in bed and not pain. A feeling of loss of control and balance are likely enhanced by visual spatial impairment. On future occasions if her daughter was not present, the care staff would swaddle her in a soft blanket and one person would hold her close and reassure her while she was being attended to.

## Case study 2: Using the DisDAT to understand distress

Alfred had dementia and cancer and was cared for in a hospice. A nurse came on night duty who had not looked after Alfred before. It was explained to her that he would sometimes get up to use the toilet at night. During the night the nurse found him sat on the edge of his bed. He was flushed, sweating and breathing rapidly. The nurse was concerned that he was experiencing an acute medical condition. The completed DisDAT documentation, however, reported that this was his usual behaviour when distressed. Understanding this, the nurse then felt confident to assist him to the bathroom to see if he needed to use the toilet. Having used the toilet, he returned to bed and comfortably settled back to sleep.

### Serial Trial Intervention (STI, Kovach *et al.* 2006)

This is a systematic approach to the management of distress when a person cannot verbally communicate their needs. Once distress is detected, the following stepwise approach is taken until distress is relieved:

- Identify and eliminate possible causes other than pain.

- Use non-pharmacological comfort measures.

- Trial the use of an analgesic or escalate the dose or regime of analgesics already taken on a regular basis.

- Refer to a specialist to assess for depression or to consider a trial of antipsychotic medication.

### Identifying and eliminating possible causes of distress (Kovach *et al.* 2006)

- Physical:

  - Are they hungry, thirsty, too hot or too cold, have they spent too long in the same position, do they need to be taken to the toilet?

  - Do they have comorbid conditions that could be causing specific symptoms to be targeted and treated?

- ○ Monitoring bowel and urine output will help identify if they are constipated or in urinary retention.

- ○ Physical examination will identify if there is skin redness, soreness, rash, broken areas or inflammation. Swellings, deformity, abdominal distension, areas of tenderness and guarding may also be detected.

- ○ Urine may be tested for signs of infection. Noisy breathing or a wheeze could indicate a chest infection. A raised temperature could indicate an infection.

- Environmental:

  - ○ The environment should be calm to avoid over-stimulation, but under-stimulation should also be avoided.

  - ○ The body language and tone of voice of the carer should be calm and reassuring.

  - ○ Sensory impairments should be addressed with glasses and hearing aids worn as appropriate.

  - ○ Orientation should be made to time and place where this is possible.

- Spiritual/psychosocial:

  - ○ Surround the person with familiar pictures, objects, perfumes, music.

  - ○ Maintain routines and identify cultural and religious practices that need to be addressed.

  - ○ Support family and friends to maintain part of the caring role.

## The use of non-pharmacological comfort measures

- Warm packs can be placed over possible areas of discomfort.

- Therapies can provide relaxation and distraction such as music and complementary therapies.

- Careful positioning of a person in the bed or chair with regular changes to their position can help to alleviate stiffness.

## DELIRIUM IN PEOPLE WITH DEMENTIA

Delirium is an acute disturbance of consciousness and cognition that develops over a short course with fluctuating symptoms (Roden and Simmonds 2014). Delirium and dementia are two of the most common causes of cognitive impairment in older people, yet their interrelation remains poorly understood (Fong *et al.* 2015). Delirium is thought to occur four to five times more often in a person with dementia. Delirium superimposed on dementia is less likely to be recognised and treated than delirium in people without dementia, as it is often attributed to a worsening of the underlying dementia. Delirium in people with dementia alerts us to the fact that there are potentially serious physical causes to be investigated and treated (Fick, Agostini and Inouye 2002).

### Characteristics of delirium

- Acute onset and fluctuations in levels of cognition and consciousness.

- Disorientation, disorganised thinking and inattention.

- Hyper-alert (hyperactive delirium) or drowsy (hypoactive delirium), or both (mixed delirium).

- Multiple potential aetiologies, rather than a specific diagnosis with a single cause.

- Potentially reversible, its presence likely indicates an underlying physical condition such as infection, dehydration, biochemical and metabolic changes, adverse reactions to medications, pain or constipation.

(Fick *et al.* 2002; NICE 2010)

## Identifying delirium in someone with dementia

To detect delirium in someone with dementia, it is important to work with family and familiar carers to understand the history of their present behaviour. Delirium is associated with an acute onset of increased and fluctuating levels of confusion, whereas the progressive decline in cognition in someone with dementia alone tends to be associated with a slower course and consciousness is not affected (Fick *et al.* 2002).

In clinical practice these distinctions are not always so clear. People with dementia are likely to have some variations in their cognitive abilities over a period of a day associated with stress or fatigue, and their confusion can appear more acute if they are in a new environment. Vascular dementia is often characterised by periods of sharp decline associated with an episode of vascular changes in the brain which could mimic an acute onset of worsening confusion, as seen in delirium.

## Managing distress in people with dementia and delirium

The guidelines for managing non-cognitive symptoms and behaviours that challenge in dementia and the guidelines for managing delirium (NICE 2010) take similar courses, reflected by the STI (Kovach *et al.* 2006).

If distressed behaviour is detected and managed according to these guidelines, the correct cause of action is likely taken regardless of whether delirium is detected. This is not surprising, as in dementia distress may occur because of pain, physical illness, anxiety, unmet needs or as a response to a confusing environment (APPG on Dementia 2008). If symptoms are not treated or needs remain unmet, they are likely to result in delirium. If the person with dementia exhibits distressed behaviour because they are thirsty and this need is not met, they may become dehydrated; if they need to go to the toilet and this is not recognised, they may become constipated or have pain that is not identified.

## Case study: Dealing with delirium in a patient with Alzheimer's

Judy is a 95-year-old widow who was diagnosed with Alzheimer's five years ago. She has lived with her son and daughter-in-law since then, who are her main carers. Judy's short-term memory is poor and she is unable to cook for herself, and needs help with washing and dressing because she cannot remember the order in which to do things. Over the years that her family has looked after her, they have identified signs of when she has a delirium caused by a chest or urine infection rather than usual dementia-related behaviour. This includes suddenly not knowing who her son and daughter-in-law are (as opposed to not remembering their names), not remembering how to walk (as opposed to slow mobility), showing fear at normal sounds (as opposed to being startled), not knowing what a knife and fork are (as opposed to not remembering how to eat), different (inappropriate) humour, not being hungry and hearing voices. When Judy shows these signs, her family talks to her GP about assessment and antibiotic-related treatment as well as what decision to make if treatment is not successful. They also put extra care plans in place to keep Judy safe (she is supervised more), dignified (she has more help with her personal hygiene) and well nourished (a variety of small, nourishing snacks which she eats with a member of the family to stimulate her to eat).

## Use of antipsychotic medication in people with dementia and delirium

At some point on their trajectory, people with dementia can experience delusions – believing things that are not true – and/ or hallucinations – seeing or hearing things that are not there (Alzheimer's Society 2012). These are also manifestations of delirium (NICE 2010). They can be frightening and frustrating experiences evoking feelings of fear, anger and anxiety. Antipsychotic medications were developed to treat people with mental health conditions such as schizophrenia, but are also effective against these psychotic symptoms of dementia and delirium (Alzheimer's Society 2012; NICE 2010).

There is a concern that in many people with dementia antipsychotics are prescribed inappropriately as a blanket first-line treatment of behaviours that challenge. Their sedative effect can mask other causes of distress such as pain, discomfort and boredom, and they can have the adverse side effects of accelerating the progression of dementia, Parkinsonism and an increased risk of falls, stroke and death (Alzheimer's Society 2012). The All Party Parliamentary Group (APPG) on Dementia (2008) recommends that a reduction in the number of inappropriate prescriptions can be achieved through staff training in person-centred care and improved care environments.

## Guidelines for using antipsychotic medication in people with dementia and delirium

- Antipsychotics should only be used to treat distress if it is severe, unresolving and cannot be de-escalated through non-pharmacological means, or if there is an immediate risk of harm to the person with dementia and others.

- If dementia is the suspected cause of the psychotic symptoms, treatment with antipsychotics should be reviewed after three months. Many people with dementia experience spontaneous resolution of the symptoms over this time.

- If delirium is suspected, a short course of antipsychotics is recommended whilst the causes of delirium are addressed.

- When antipsychotic medications are advocated, there needs to be a discussion with the person with dementia if this is possible and their family, to highlight the benefits and risks of the treatment.

(NICE 2010)

## Delirium and palliative care

The guidelines on using antipsychotic medication in dementia and delirium do not cover issues specific to end of life care. When the person moves into the dying phase, decisions against invasive corrective treatment are usually taken and emphasis is placed on symptom management and comfort. When infection, dehydration, malnutrition, anaemia and electrolyte imbalances relating to the dying process are no longer reversible, delirium can dominate the clinical picture. It could be argued that in the dying phase there needs to be a lower threshold for using antipsychotic medication to alleviate even moderate levels of distress that is unresolved by other means (Treloar *et al.* 2010).

## Terminal restlessness

This is delirium that occurs in the last days to hours of life, exacerbated by the progressive shutdown of multiple body systems. It may appear as involuntary muscle twitching, fidgeting, tossing and turning, yelling or moaning, and occurs in 25–85 per cent of terminally ill patients (Lawlor, Fainsinger and Bruera 2000). It can be a distressing experience for the patient and also their loved ones, for whom this memory can interfere with their grieving process (Travis *et al.* 2001). It requires urgent pharmacological management with antipsychotics and/or benzodiazepines for their anxiolytic and sedative properties (Twycross and Wilcock 2001).

## WHEN A PERSON WITH DEMENTIA STOPS EATING AND DRINKING

When someone with dementia experiences difficulties eating and drinking, it is important to explore other causes before assuming it is because of the severity of their dementia (Regnard and Huntley 2006).

## Possible causes

- *Sore mouth:* Thrush, tooth decay, gum disease or poor-fitting dentures. Thrush is easily treated with oral preparations, and while dental treatments may be too distressing, more simple remedies may be employed such as denture-fixing cream, local analgesic gels, systemic analgesics and avoiding acidic or hot or cold foods.

- *Environment:* For most people the experience of eating and drinking is sociable. The environment should be kept conducive and non-hurried, and distractions avoided. Think about the layout of food on the plate and contrasting coloured crockery so that food can be distinguished on the plate.

- *Taste changes or difficulty recognising food:* There may be a preference for strong-tasting foods, sweet foods or finger foods, and these preferences may vary from day to day.

- *Depression:* This may be indicated by loss of interest in food and poor appetite.

- *Nausea:* This may be a result of a physical illness, constipation or the side effects of medication.

## Loss of ability to coordinate chewing and swallowing in end-stage dementia

When these difficulties occur, small amounts of soft food and thickened fluids should be offered at frequent intervals with the person sat upright. There may come a time when they are no longer able to eat and drink because the severity of the swallowing difficulty causes them to cough and choke and they become distressed. Aspiration pneumonia is the likely outcome caused by small amounts of food or liquids entering the lungs (Summersall and Wight 2004).

Enteral feeding is often a considered solution, but research shows that it does not prevent weight loss or aspiration pneumonia in people with advanced dementia (Finucane, Christmas and Travis 1999). In advanced stages of a progressive disease, anorexia and cachexia are a result of an altered state of metabolism causing involuntary accelerated weight loss, including muscle loss, regardless of calorie intake (Fabbro, Dalal and Bruera 2006). The presence of a feeding tube does not prevent aspiration of saliva, and there is a greater risk of reflux and aspiration of gastric contents (Finucane *et al.* 1999).

Some of the burdens associated with enteral feeding have been reported as:

- losing the social aspect and pleasure of eating

- the need for admission to hospital

- abdominal discomfort and nausea

- diarrhoea

- risk of infection at the tube site

- risk of the tube leaking, and blocking of the tube

- risk of the tube being pulled out

- increased urine and stool output in someone who is incontinent.

(Gillick 2000)

According to NICE (2010) guidance, people with dementia should be encouraged to eat and drink by mouth for as long as possible, and enteral feeding should generally not be used in people with severe dementia except in circumstances where dysphagia is considered to be a transient phenomenon rather than a manifestation of the severity of the dementia.

## Case study: Exploring issues around eating difficulties

June has end-stage Alzheimer's disease and is cared for in a nursing home. She now has very little appetite but enjoys a few spoons of her favourite ice cream, which Jim, her husband, brings for her. If you try and get her to eat more, she becomes distressed. Over the last few months she has lost a considerable amount of weight. Jim is very happy with the care she receives and does not want anything that distresses her.

Her daughter Susan had not been able to visit for a while, and is shocked to see her mother looking so frail and thin. She confronts the nursing home staff, saying that they have not been providing adequate care for her mother. She is aware that another lady in the home is fed artificially by a feeding tube, and she asks why the same is not done for her mother.

It is explained to Susan that for some people swallowing difficulties might be a temporary condition, as a result of a stroke, for example, and enteral feeding is used to support their recovery. June's poor appetite and swallowing difficulties are due to the irreversible progression of her dementia. In this case the distress and burden of having a feeding tube would likely reduce the quality of her end of life.

## MEDICATIONS AT THE END OF LIFE FOR PEOPLE WITH DEMENTIA

When the end of life phase is reached, medications should be rationalised and limited to those required for managing symptoms of pain and discomfort such as nausea and breathlessness. These include analgesics, antiemetics, and anxiolytic, antipsychotic and anticholinergic drugs.

### Use of antibiotics

Although the medical treatment of infection in advanced dementia does not limit the progression of dementia, antibiotics may improve the symptoms of fever, pain and breathlessness associated with infection. The decision to treat with antibiotics should be made on an individual basis and take into account the person's wishes, their ability to swallow, tolerate or accept oral medication, how effective this has been previously, the risk of iatrogenic illness and the need for hospitalisation (NICE 2010).

## Symptom management and medication

It is often helpful for clinical teams (from all disciplines, including palliative care, elderly care, and primary and secondary care) and carers/family to discuss together symptom control goals and management.

Consider the following:

- A person with dementia in your care requires regular analgesics, but sometimes will not take them. How would you address this situation?

If they have capacity to make the decision to refuse analgesics, it is important to ensure they understand the benefits of taking regular analgesics. If it is assessed that they do not have capacity to make this decision, a meeting with healthcare professionals and family carers may be held to discuss ways of acting in the person's best interests. Alternative non-oral preparations may be felt to be more appropriate.

- If a person is no longer able to swallow oral analgesics, what are the alternative methods of giving analgesia?

Analgesic gels can be applied to areas of localised pain. Transdermal patches may be used to give systemic relief. These are applied to the patient's skin and the analgesia is absorbed through the skin into the bloodstream to give a continuous dose. Transdermal patches are not recommended for unstable pain as their half-life makes it difficult to titrate pain control effectively. In the terminal stages subcutaneous injections or a subcutaneous infusion may be used.[2]


## Syringe pumps

A syringe pump is a portable battery-operated device that delivers medication subcutaneously over a continuous 24-hour period for patients who are unable to take oral medication. The aim of the syringe pump is to control symptoms, not to shorten life. The patient may have functional swallowing

---

2    The text here has been used with the permission of BUPA (2010).

difficulties, intractable nausea and vomiting, be unable to understand and rationalise the need to take the medication or they may be semi-conscious. A syringe pump is not just for analgesic administration, but enables a combination of drugs for symptom relief to be administered in one infusion.

## Subcutaneous injections

It is not always possible to implement the use of a syringe pump. This may be because there is a lack of equipment or trained staff, or the patient with dementia and confusion may pull it out. Subcutaneous injections are an alternative means of administering a range of symptom management drugs. Injections are administered through a fine-bore needle at a 45-degree angle into the subcutaneous tissue just below the skin. They are less invasive and less painful than intramuscular injections. They may be used regularly or 'as required'.

## PROVIDING 'COMFORT MEASURES' AT THE END OF LIFE

Aggressive medical treatment for acute infection, malnutrition and dehydration does not limit dementia progression in advanced stages (Hurley, Volicer and Volicer 1996; Meier *et al.* 2001; Mitchell, Kieley and Hamel 2004). At this stage an approach that focuses on managing symptoms and promoting comfort while avoiding the distress of invasive investigations and medical treatments will enhance the quality of end of life. Determining the end stage, which is often protracted and complicated by the existence of other comorbidities, along with the person's lack of capacity to make complex decisions, poses problems in deciding when to withhold active treatment.

The Gold Standards Framework (GSF) (Thomas 2010), outlined earlier in Chapter 1, encourages practitioners to review their treatment decision-making. It includes guidance on prognostic indicators for people with dementia. It is not intended to be prescriptive, and decisions about care should not be based on survival alone. The burden and benefits of various treatments, the person's quality of life and degree of suffering and their known or perceived wishes should all be taken into account (Mental Capacity Act 2005).

When the person with dementia is no longer able to engage in discussions, the ultimate responsibility for decisions in the best interests of the person about end of life care rests with the family and healthcare professionals. The dilemmas and stress experienced by family carers at this time are discussed later, in Chapter 4. They often feel unprepared for this role of proxy decision-maker. They wish to preserve the dignity and comfort of their relative but have difficulty incorporating comfort care into specific plans (Forbes, Bern-Klug and Gessert 2000).

It is valuable to take into account previously expressed wishes or family/carers' beliefs about how the person likes to be physically cared for. In addition, consider the following:

- Nurse the person on a pressure-relieving mattress to prevent pressure sores.

- Maintain a comfortable temperature. A fan may help if they have a fever or are breathless.

- Monitor urinary output and bowel motions. A urinary catheter is normally avoided due to the risk of delirium, but may be required at this stage if there is retention of urine. Reduced fluid and dietary intake, immobility and analgesic medications increase the risks of constipation, and laxatives or suppositories may be required.

- Maintain skin care with moisturising and barrier creams.

- Ensure good oral hygiene. When the person is no longer eating and drinking, keep the mouth moist with water on a small sponge, or use artificial saliva. Apply lip balm to keep their lips moist.

- Complementary therapy such as gentle hand massage and aromatherapy oils can provide relaxation.

- Keep the environment peaceful and surround the person with familiar objects, pictures and music, if they enjoy it. Encourage family members to sit with them and communicate through non-verbal methods of touch, tone of voice and facial expressions.

- Maintain continuity of staff involved in the person's care and encourage relatives to tell their life stories to help the staff connect with who they are.

- Adhere to and support the family in maintaining beliefs and customs, and record details of care required at the time of death.[3]

## Key points

- Symptom assessment needs to be holistic and involve the family and familiar carers. Information should be gathered using multiple methods and a range of sources to provide a comprehensive picture of the person's experience.

- Pain assessment for people with dementia who can report their pain should involve a mixture of supportive communication techniques, self-report assessment tools in a visual format, and behavioural observation tools.

- For people with advanced dementia and severe communication difficulties, behavioural observation tools are used to identify when they are distressed. A systematic approach is then needed to determine the cause of their distress, which may be physical, psychosocial or spiritual.

- Delirium in people with dementia alerts us to the fact that there are potentially serious physical causes to be investigated and treated.

---

3   Used with permission of BUPA 2010.

- The Serial Trial Intervention (STI) is an approach that can be followed to manage distress in someone with dementia and someone with delirium.
- Antipsychotic medication is considered as a last resort for managing distress in dementia and delirium if it remains severe and unresolved by other measures. Owing to the risks of adverse side effects, these should be reviewed regularly and stopped after an appropriate period of symptom resolution.
- In the dying phase, delirium can dominate the clinical picture as it may not be possible to address all the reversible causes. In this situation it could be argued that antipsychotic medication may be used to treat even moderate levels of distress that are not resolved by other means.
- Terminal agitation is intractable delirium in the last days to hours of life that requires pharmacological management with antipsychotics and/or benzodiazepines.
- People with dementia should be encouraged to eat and drink for as long as possible, and enteral feeding should generally not be used in people with advanced dementia, except in circumstances where dysphagia is a transient phenomenon rather than a manifestation of the severity of the dementia.
- Aggressive medical treatment for acute infection, malnutrition and dehydration does not limit dementia progression in advanced stages. A palliative care approach can avoid the distress of invasive investigations and medical treatments at the end of life.
- Medications at the end of life should be rationalised and limited to those required for managing symptoms of pain and discomfort.
- There are alternative routes for administering symptom management medication for people who are unable to swallow, tolerate or understand the need to take oral medication.

Chapter 3

# Emotional Wellbeing and Dignity

**Learning outcomes**

By the end of this chapter you will be able to:

- Identify the universal needs of people at the end of life.

- Consider those needs specifically in the context of people with dementia.

- Identify barriers to enhancing dignity and emotional wellbeing for people with dementia.

- Identify strategies to minimise those barriers to dignity.

- Identify interventions that can enhance emotional wellbeing for people with dementia approaching the end of life.

- Consider how stimulation of each of the five senses can be used as an intervention to promote emotional wellbeing.

- Identify the dying phase, and consider how a person's needs change as they enter the last days of life.

All humans have fundamental and universal needs throughout life, perhaps most significantly felt during times of vulnerability. Abraham Maslow observed 80 years ago that these needs exist as a hierarchy (Robinson *et al.* 2012; see also Figure 3.1), and that people are unable to achieve higher level needs (such as self-actualisation, relationships or connection) unless lower level needs (such as homeostasis, eating, sleeping and so on) are met. As dementia advances, it is easy to assume that higher level needs become less important and care is aimed at focusing predominantly on the physical aspects of people's needs. However, people with advanced dementia are known to express a range of emotions in response to differing situations (Deno *et al.* 2012); therefore, despite the challenges inherent in interpreting and communicating responses, there is a clear need to integrate emotional awareness into the care of people dying with dementia.

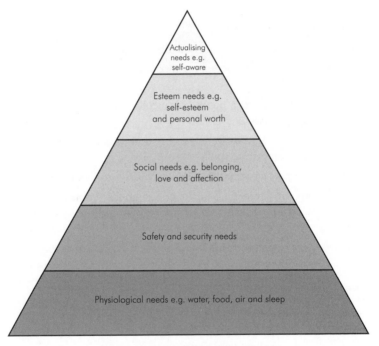

Figure 3.1 Maslow's hierarchy of needs
*Source: Maslow (1943)*

This chapter explores the psychosocial needs of people with dementia at the end of life. It begins with a brief review of what is known about general and universal human needs as death approaches. This is then applied to the care of people who have diminishing verbal and cognitive capacity. In the presence of communication difficulties, non-verbal communication and the maintenance of a safe, compassionate care environment become increasingly significant. The concept of dignity as it applies to people with dementia is briefly discussed. We then explore some ways in which this might be achieved in the various settings in which people with dementia spend the last days of their lives, by considering the senses as a vehicle for connection, and discussing the process of care planning and the delivery of individualised care. A range of interventions is presented. Finally, some examples of dilemmas of care in relation to maintaining dignity and emotional wellbeing are considered.

Before we begin to explore how we might maintain and support dignity in people with dementia at the end of life, it is important that we obtain a clarification of what we understand by 'dignity'. Dignity is a term that is widely used in ethical, professional, philosophical and legal discourse. Aristotle wrote extensively on the notion that humans are of value or worth because they possess certain characteristics. These ideas were further developed by Immanuel Kant, who proposed that human beings possess dignity on account of the fact that they are rational, autonomous creatures with intrinsic value *who can pursue and determine their own ends* (Kant 1967). In other words, the ability to determine one's actions is the way in which human beings obtain dignity.

This is somewhat troublesome as a concept, as it implies that a human being who is not rational or able to determine his or her own ends will somehow lack dignity as a direct consequence. Kant's concept of dignity was subsequently developed into *Menschenwürde*, a term which refers to dignity being inherent and not reliant on the person having rationality (Nordenfelt 2004, pp.83–89).

Thus a person with dementia by their very existence possesses inherent dignity that can either be enhanced or diminished by the environment in which they exist. It has been suggested that dignity can be defined by examining the interplay between the circumstances in which we find ourselves and our capabilities (Shotton and Seedhouse 1998). This definition points towards situations where we find ourselves lacking dignity, and observes the common features of such situations, such as where we feel inadequate, incompetent, foolish or vulnerable. It is the last feature that applies particularly to people with dementia. As reported by Andersen *et al.*, Bayer undertook an extensive focus group and interview study in six European countries in order to identify what older people mean by dignity (Andersen *et al.* 2011). Three themes were identified: respect and recognition, participation, and involvement. Participants reported that they felt dignity was enhanced through communication, privacy, maintenance of personal identity and minimising vulnerability. Particularly at the end of life, people with dementia become vulnerable. This notion of vulnerability is poignantly summarised in an extract from a carer's account of her grandfather:

> Human vulnerability is made no more terrifyingly visible than in those people with dementia. My grandfather – the pilot, the physician, the jazz musician – now cannot tie his own shoes. This might be you or me, tomorrow or in 20 years. (Harper 2013)

Tom Kitwood advocated the notion of personhood in dementia care (Kitwood 1997). This was not a new concept; philosophers such as J.P. Moreland proposed that all beings (entities) possess an essence, and it is this essence which gives a being unity, which enables them to maintain identity through change. It is beyond the remit of this book to enter into an epistemological discussion over whether a person with advanced dementia is, in fact, the same person they were prior to their dementia. There does seem to be consensus that wellbeing in dementia is firmly associated with interventions that promote recognition of the person within, whether or not that person is able to be understood. For example, a recent integrative review by Johnston and Narayanasamy (2016) reported that, generally, personhood aspects of interventions were well reported, but further research is required to explore the legacy potential of psychosocial interventions for people with dementia.

Kitwood's contribution to the field was to identify that many of the ways in which dementia care goes wrong is attributable to actions which, consciously or unconsciously, adversely affect the personhood of the person with dementia. He argued that viewing people with dementia in purely medical terms has led to them being treated as objects, without identities or subjectivity. He highlights the importance of biography and interaction as being ways to facilitate the recognition of personhood, and argues that the quality of care is highly dependent on this fundamental shift in attitude.

A literature review by Gallagher *et al.* (2008) explored research with elderly patients and their relatives related to aspects of care felt to promote or diminish dignity. They identified four key themes:

- *Environment of care:* The context in which care is given, and the conditions that can lead to people being treated with dignity. For example, mixed-sex facilities are considered to be a potential violation of dignity for many people.

- *Staff attitudes and behaviour:* The way in which individuals respond to people with dementia. For example, 'not being seen' was considered to be a violation of dignity, as demonstrated when staff talked over or disregarded the view of a person with dementia.

- *Culture of care:* The shared beliefs and values that prevail in a given care setting. For example, valuing the place of sensory stimulation and fostering a sense of purpose are considered to improve subjective wellbeing. The philosophy of a particular care setting will dictate how the people with dementia are viewed as part of that setting.

- *Specific care activities:* Bathing, toileting, feeding and other activities of living. For example, access to lavatory facilities, being enabled to access these rather than risking incontinence, or being made to wear continence pads to make things easier for care staff.

In the last weeks and months of life, the needs of a person with dementia are likely to change. Kitwood identifies that people with dementia possess six psychological needs: *attachment, love, comfort, identity, inclusion* and *occupation*. We now explore how these needs can be illustrated in a number of ways and how dignity can be maintained or diminished by how a person with dementia is treated at the end of life.

## COMFORT

Comfort is one of the main concerns that people express when considering their needs as death approaches. *The Oxford Dictionary* defines 'comfort' as either (1) a 'state of physical ease and freedom from pain or constraint', or (2) 'consolation for grief or anxiety' (Sykes 1979). Maintaining physical and emotional comfort forms the mainstay of the palliative approach to care, alleviating suffering rather than attempting to prolong life.

The literature suggests that physical comfort and symptom control are less prominent concerns for people than psychosocial care (Black 2011). However, a brief review of the evidence on end of life care reveals a vast imbalance between research on physical comfort measures such as pain, and non-physical issues such as loneliness, boredom, isolation or anxiety. This mismatch may present carers and families with the perception that the priority of care is the management of physical 'problems', which can lead to a culture of problem identification and task-focused interventions. Of course, relating this back to Maslow's hierarchy, we can see that in many ways the tendency of health and social care professionals to meet basic needs first is not misguided. Indeed, a person who is hungry or cold is hardly likely to engage in therapeutic interventions aimed at improving a sense of belonging or achievement. However, an exclusive focus on physical needs to the exclusion of non-physical needs means that care is incomplete.

### Case study: Exploring how to support carers

Rodney has osteoarthritis and advanced Alzheimer's disease. He is cared for by his wife, Carol, with support from Social Services. His mobility has deteriorated significantly, and his impaired coordination due to Alzheimer's, combined with his poor mobility resulting from arthritis, have led to his being bed- and chair-bound for most of the time. Carol has found caring increasingly difficult, and when the carers visit one day she bursts into tears and tells them that, while trying to read to him from his favourite series of magazines, he had an uncharacteristically aggressive outburst, telling her to go away and leave him alone.

One way of contextualising this scenario is to consider the impact of Rodney's physical condition on his emotional state. It may be that pain from his arthritis is causing him to feel distressed, and that Carol's compassionate and well-meaning attempts to engage him in a pastime that he has drawn much enjoyment from in the past may not be appropriate at this point. The carers could approach this by considering interventions that may help with his physical comfort, by explaining to Carol the concepts inherent in Maslow's hierarchy. Once Rodney is physically comfortable, he may be more relaxed just sitting.

Many of the psychological features of dementia may become more acute as the end of life approaches. Patients may experience delusions, hallucinations or paranoia. Behaviour may indicate depression or aggression. Unfortunately, the evidence demonstrates high rates of antipsychotic prescriptions to manage such problems (Connolly, Sampson and Purandare 2012), with the result that quality of life may be further impaired. This has been discussed earlier in Chapter 2, but it is important to note that the consequences of unnecessary sedation are far-reaching, impacting on the family and carers as well as the patient.

So how can problems be managed without resorting to medication? Management of distress needs to follow from an accurate assessment of potential causes. Ask the following questions:

- Is this behaviour out of character?

- Has there been a recent onset of behaviour change?

- Recent changes in environment (new staff, visit from family member, change in food)?
- What else could it indicate?
  - pain, e.g. contractures, arthritis, decubitus ulcer
  - constipation
  - urinary retention
  - infection
  - spiritual/existential distress.

## LOVE

At the core of the person with dementia, spiritual matters remain pervasively in the background. They offer potential pathways for connections amidst the fear and vagueness of what cannot be reached, spoken about, or validated by others who have no idea as to who the person *really is inside* or once was. (Lawrence 2003)

Studies show that patients with dementia typically receive significantly fewer spiritual or religious interventions than patients without cognitive impairment (Ruddon 2010). Spiritual care is an elusive term and may or may not include religious needs, and is important throughout the patient's journey regardless of stage of life. However, death is a profoundly significant event for all humans, regardless of religious or spiritual beliefs, and the importance of spiritual support at the end of life has been demonstrated in a range of studies (see, for example, Gijsberts et al. 2013; Ødbehr et al. 2015; Puchalski et al. 2006; van der Steen et al. 2013).

A common thread in most discussions about spirituality in healthcare relates to the notion of connectedness. Those who are able to communicate can create and sustain connectedness with others and with their environment through the interpretive looking glass of their cultural conditioning. For those who are unable to do so, connectedness can be created in other ways:

- Fostering a sense of identity.

- Encouraging a sense of belonging and security.

- Giving and receiving affection.

- Respecting the need for space, privacy and dignity.

- Listening and responding, with or without words, with patience and respect.

- Empowering/facilitating occupation and participation.

- Providing special occasions and making every day special.

- Being alongside in times of unsupportable distress.

- Helping to maintain faith practices and contact with faith groups.

- Welcoming and affirming the contribution which people with dementia can make to the spiritual life of others.

## Case study: Considering cultural, religious and spiritual concerns

Aman is originally from India and is a practising Sikh. He has attended his local temple ever since he moved to the UK 30 years ago. He is a widower, and has four children who visit regularly. He has been admitted to hospital with an infected grade 4 pressure sore, which has led to him requiring intravenous antibiotics. The wound does not appear to be improving despite this treatment, and the multidisciplinary team are in agreement that he is likely to be approaching the end of life. Karen, a staff nurse on the medical ward, asks Aman's son Charandev whether there might be anyone from the temple who he thinks Aman would like to have visit him. Charandev feels that Aman would not want visitors, as he believes his father is distressed by the odour from his wound, and asks instead if he can bring in a CD of spiritual songs for his father to listen to. Karen is concerned about this, as Aman is in a shared bay, but speaks to the ward sister, who agrees that since he is at the end of life it would be preferable in any case to move him to a side room. Unfortunately, none are available, so the nurse suggests to Charandev that he brings some headphones, which he does. Aman is noted by staff to visibly relax when the music is played, and they set the CD player to play continuously. Karen comments on how surprised she is by how comfortable Aman appears, despite the severe wound and their assumptions that he would have significant physical pain. Charandev believes that his father's faith provided comfort to the extent that his physical condition did not seem to cause him distress. He died with the music still playing in his ears, four days later, with his family at his bedside, behind curtains, on a shared hospital ward. Later, Charandev tells Karen that Aman means 'peaceful one'. Karen is deeply affected by this experience.

## IDENTITY

The *End of Life Care Strategy* suggests that, for many, the notion of a good death includes being treated as an individual, with dignity and respect, being without pain and other symptoms, being in familiar surroundings, and being in the company of close family and friends (DH 2008a). This is the case for people with or without a diagnosis of dementia.

The dying process may involve a period of time where the person becomes unable to communicate their thoughts and needs. For people with cancer, this period may be short – perhaps hours or days. For those dying with dementia this terminal stage follows a gradual and prolonged decline in communicative ability. If the person is being cared for in a familiar environment, by people with whom they have a relationship, maintenance of their individual personhood is less challenging than if they are admitted to hospital or hospice, finding themselves in an unfamiliar environment with carers who may know little more than their name, diagnosis and date of birth.

## Case study: Ensuring person-centred approach includes body image

Monty was a renowned lecturer in philosophy who lived with his partner, Bert, in a cottage in remote Perthshire. When he first developed dementia, Bert cared for him at home. Monty was admitted to a care home in a nearby town when Bert developed pneumonia and subsequently died. They had no other relatives and their friends were scattered all over the world, with minimal contact in recent years. When he arrived, Monty was in a dishevelled state. He had a beard and his hair was long and tangled. Staff were distressed to discover that Monty had scabies, and they promptly administered topical treatment for his hair and skin. He was shaved and shampooed, and his threadbare clothes were replaced with a new pair of trousers and a shirt. A domiciliary hairdresser visited and cut Monty's hair short, giving him a neat short back and sides that is popular with men of his age. Staff felt that they had worked well together, and although it had been 'a bit of a battle' giving Monty a bath, he 'must feel better for it'. Monty was deeply distressed by the experience, however, and remained curled up in bed for several days with his eyes squeezed tightly closed, resisting with violence any attempts to touch him physically.

Of course, we are not advocating that Monty should be left, parasites and all, in the state in which he was admitted. However, this illustrates an important point. None of the care staff had any idea which aspects of his physical appearance Monty was attached to, and which were the result of recent weeks of inadvertent neglect by his ailing partner. We do not know what value he ascribed to his beard, to his long hair, or indeed to the clothes that had been thrown away. As Monty was not able to communicate verbally, staff had to respond by grooming him in the way in which they assumed he would want. It may have been less traumatic for Monty had this been done gradually, perhaps paying close attention to how he responded to various interventions. Possibly cleanliness and treating his infestation could have been prioritised. Perhaps staff could have obtained from his home some photographs of his appearance earlier in life? Or as he had been a lecturer, could they have contacted his institution to see whether there were any institutional records, perhaps photographic records, of him in publications? Furthermore, although we do not know the extent of Monty's awareness of his surroundings, the grief arising from the sudden unexplained absence of Bert may also be having a profound influence on his wellbeing.

## Case study: Challenges of caring for someone whose wishes and preferences are unknown

Edna is admitted to hospital with a chest infection. She has been living in a care home for six years and has become progressively more withdrawn and unable to communicate, with a period of rapid decline over recent months. On arrival she is semi-comatose, making soft moaning sounds, and pyrexial. The admitting nurse places a name band on her wrist, as well as a red one to identify her allergy to penicillin. Her temperature is taken and she is changed from her skirt and jumper into a hospital gown, and put into bed in a bay of four patients. A cannula is sited in her arm, and an infusion of saline is commenced. The nurse perceives that she is unable to respond, so does not speak to her whilst performing these tasks. Given her poor physical state, the nurse expects that there will not be a problem with this patient wandering around the ward. Secretly she feels relieved; patients with dementia can often be challenging to care for on the busy medical ward. Edna appears unaware of the nursing interventions, occasionally screwing up her face or making quiet sounds.

How much do the staff know about Edna's wishes? Has she been admitted with notes from the nursing home outlining her preferences with regards to her personal hygiene? She might prefer the use of a particular face cream, the scent of which makes her feel at home. How is her bed positioned in the ward in relation to light? Is she in the full glare of fluorescent lighting and unable to turn her face away? What are the smells and sounds she is exposed to usually in the care home she lives in?

McCormack (2003) suggests that person-centredness in practice is exemplified by authentic consciousness, an awareness of a person's fundamental values. Making the effort to find out who this person has been, and what their familiar world looks and feels like, may be a key way to find the point of connection between them and the outside world.

## OCCUPATION AND INCLUSION

A review of the literature exploring the needs of people at the end of life identified the maintenance of normality as a key concern across a range of populations (Black 2011), although none of the identified research related specifically to people with dementia (presumably due to methodological difficulties in obtaining this information directly). However, continuing the imperative to maintain personhood is vital in people with dementia. The need for normality is doubtless still there, even though the shape of that 'normality' may have altered significantly over the years of having dementia.

## Case study: Preserving personhood

Maureen had been a matron of a nursing home for over 40 years. When she was diagnosed with dementia, she was unable to remain at home as she was widowed, and her children lived abroad. She was admitted to a local care home. It was noticed that she took great interest in the conversations that the nurses and care staff had, whether in the lounge, the nurses' station or by the bedside. Whilst still mobile, she had a tendency to run her fingers across surfaces and check them for dust. She would also frequently visit other residents in their rooms and talk softly but unintelligibly to them. Initially, staff found this difficult to manage, trying to discourage her and distract her with other activities. Following a visit from her daughter where they were able to gain more insight into her life as a nursing home matron, they realised that this was a fundamental part of her identity. They produced a care plan in which they provided her with opportunities to clean small ornaments, and rearrange files of blank paper. They ensured that she sat with residents who were happy to be talked to. In this way, normality was sustained, albeit in an artificial way. When her condition meant it was difficult for her to leave her bedroom, staff ensured that she still had opportunities to feel involved in the life of the nursing home, by using a hoist and wheelchair to sit her in the busy lounge, among the sounds and sights with which she had become familiar. Even though she spent most of her time sleeping in the chair, staff felt that she was happier and calmer being at the centre of things than hidden away in the quiet of her bedroom.

As people become closer to death, the interactions they have with professional carers may take on increasingly task-orientated characteristics. Routine turns to relieve pressure areas, mouth care, administration of medications and so on replace the social interactions that may bring comfort in a different and intangible way.

## Case study: Thinking about 'being with' and not just 'doing for'

Kelly is a first-year student nurse on a care of the elderly ward. The ward is busy and noisy, and her mentor is frequently occupied with administering medications and caring for patients who are confused or anxious. Kelly is looking after Raymond, who is a bed-bound patient with advanced vascular dementia, his bed positioned at the far end of the ward from the nursing station. He is dying. Kelly has helped the healthcare support workers to give him a bed bath that morning. They then move on to 'do cares' on the next patient. Kelly decides to sit with Raymond for a while. Her supernumary status means she is not counted in the ward staffing numbers, so she is able to take this opportunity that paid staff may not. She sits beside the bed on a chair and puts her hand on his. She tells him what it is like being a student nurse, about her grandma who suffered from dementia, about the holiday she was looking forward to that summer. After talking for ten minutes or so, she goes to find out how to help staff with the other patients.

It is important to encourage students to spend time with people dying with dementia. It is a privilege to witness this profound life process, and this may enhance their learning experience immeasurably. It is also important to identify how many staff interventions are task-focused, and how many are intended to connect with the person. If there is an imbalance, consider developing non-task-orientated interventions as an individual care plan.

## CONNECTING WITH THE DYING PERSON

People with dementia may be unable to communicate their needs directly. However, they remain in possession of all of their physical senses, albeit sometimes in an altered or diminished capacity. Regardless of the care setting, it is possible to create a meaningful environment that respects the person within. As well as maintaining physical comfort, the health and social care professional can play an important part in the creation of opportunities for connection and compassionate care using a variety of sense modalities. The dying phase is a time to transcend traditional modes of care, such as task-focused interventions, and create a compassionate and comforting environment in which somebody can experience a peaceful death.

## Touch

From early in gestation, humans begin to respond to tactile stimulation (Gethin 2012). Touch serves two purposes: it warns us of imminent danger (as in the example of warmth increasing to uncomfortable heat), or it communicates pleasure and connection (as in sensual touch) (Liu, Guarino and Lopez 2011). This human capacity is thought to exist right until the end of life. The touching of different body parts conveys different messages. Because cultural, personality and historical factors all converge to create different meanings for different forms of tactile contact, this is another context where knowledge of the individual person is key. What is seen as pleasant, platonic interaction by one individual may be perceived as invasive and unpleasant by somebody else. There is evidence that certain parts of the brain – namely, the orbitofrontal cortex – respond specifically to pleasant touch (Catt *et al.* 2005). This part of the brain is older, in evolutionary terms, than the somatosensory cortex that is associated with the localisation of painful touch stimuli. This suggests that the evolution of pleasure in response to stimuli is primal (Hardy 2012).

Somebody with dementia may only experience touch in the context of being washed and changed, or undergoing medical interventions or procedures. Often the human aspect of connectedness, which we convey through touch, is lacking. In some instances, if this has been the case for a long period of time, suddenly being touched may cause agitation or distress, since it will be unfamiliar.

## Scent

Do certain odours evoke a sense of earlier life? Perhaps he worked in a bakery? Or was she a hairdresser? Or did they live near a brewery or farmyard? All of these may be potentially fruitful avenues of communication and connection.

The use of aromatherapy in dementia is receiving increased attention in the research literature. A Korean study has identified that use of lavender oil aromatherapy significantly reduces aggression in elderly patients with dementia (Michaelson, Knight and Fink 2002). Studies on populations without dementia have identified improved sleep patterns following aromatherapy treatment (Maben, Latter and Macleod Clark 2006). Although there is little research on the use of other aromatherapy oils, many of the studies found improvement in affect and mood and reduced aggression through massage alone, in the absence of scented oils, reinforcing the importance of therapeutic touch. Despite methodological issues with some of these research studies, the use of aromatherapy is known to be safe and may be helpful in creating a calm and nurturing atmosphere for patients.

## Sound

Did this person enjoy music or play an instrument when they were younger? Or do they, perhaps, have a favourite artist or genre? Again, paying attention to the individual is of paramount importance here. A research project identified a possible reduction in depressive symptoms in people with dementia who participated in reminiscence-focused music sessions (Ashida 2000), although admittedly this study was small scale and was undertaken with dementia patients who were not necessarily in the last year of life and may have still had some communicative ability. Paul Robertson, however, believes that the brain's auditory system remains intact and responsive to music and sounds long after other parts of neurological functioning have ceased (Robertson 2001).

## Sight

There are numerous changes with sight that are associated with advancing dementia (Connor *et al.* 2004). These include difficulties perceiving in three dimensions, a need for brighter lighting, reduced contrast between colours and shrinking peripheral vision. It has been argued that the behaviours associated with 'sundowning' (increased agitation in the early evenings) are related to trouble with glare and shadows. Anyone attempting to create a calm space around the dying person needs to take this into account. For example, avoid placing objects of visual interest in locations where they occupy peripheral vision only, particularly if contractures or weakness make it difficult for the person to turn their face. Quality and intensity of light is also an important consideration. Older people may be more sensitive to glare, and bright light is known to affect the quality and quantity of sleep (Dewing 2009). Avoid glare of sunlight directly on the person's face, and set up interesting images and objects with bright colours and contrast.

### Case study: Understanding and allowing emotional expression

Consider the case of Mike and his dad, Sid. Sid is clearly expressing distress, although it is unclear what the source of this distress is. It may be that he has a profound recognition of his son but his presence makes him aware of his inability to communicate. Staff may have missed an opportunity here. The expression of distress is clear evidence of Sid's residual capacity to feel and to express emotions. Staff could have made the most of Mike's statement that he 'felt silly' just talking to Sid in the absence of any meaningful responses. He may have felt reassured by receiving an explanation that just because his dad does not reply does not mean he does not derive comfort from his presence. Furthermore, some people perceive tears to be an expression of distress and to be avoided. However, it is generally acknowledged within the psychological literature that crying has an important function in the expression and catharsis of emotion. Indeed, in the absence of his being able to communicate emotions in any other way, Sid's tears could be reconceptualised as a profound source of connection with Mike. Mike may be reassured through the explanation that Sid feels comfortable enough in his presence to express himself through tears.

## Case study: Being aware of the person in the broader context of their family

Consider the case of Badriya. Badriya moved to the UK in the 1980s to marry Hafeez. They have two daughters – Seeta is married and has a child with cerebral palsy, and Rashida is studying at the local university. Hafeez is self-employed and works long hours. Badriya has numerous medical problems, including vascular dementia and heart failure. She has a leg ulcer which is proving difficult to heal, partly because of her poor circulation and oedema, and partly because she is inclined to try to remove dressings that the nurses apply. The visiting district nursing staff have the perception that she has a large and supportive family and have therefore not been particularly proactive in acknowledging the difficulties that Badriya's family are experiencing trying to keep her safe and at home. Hafeez believes that home is the right place for her to be, despite increasingly complex care requirements. However, there does seem to be some family tension with regards to how to facilitate this care arrangement.

It may be that the nurses need to listen carefully to each family member's concerns in a group discussion, and to highlight in a non-judgemental way the tensions that exist. A compromise may be possible; for example, could a sitter be obtained for part of the time? Could an occasional respite admission help? What are the issues relating to the wound dressing – does Hafeez understand the reasons for her wound not healing or is he blaming the treatment? Careful explanation and empathy are required here. It is interesting to note that people with dementia who are from minority ethnic groups appear to receive significantly fewer supportive interventions at the end of life (Connolly, Sampson and Purandare 2012).

## Case study: Assessing behavioural symptoms

Staff on the ward looking after Harry are limited in how able they are to accurately assess how much of his disturbed behaviour relates to his current state of physical frailty and how much relates to his disorientation at having been so unwell and then coming round to find himself in an unfamiliar environment. Changes in behaviour are far harder to detect if you do not have prior knowledge of the way in which people previously expressed themselves. It may be helpful for staff to liaise with Harry's usual carers to describe his current behaviour in order to try to ascertain whether there may be underlying issues that are contributing to his distress. The Alzheimer's Society produces a guide for carers[1] that prompts them to observe behaviours that may indicate some underlying distress. The National Council for Palliative Care also produces a useful guide for pain and distress (NCPC 2012). The registrar suggests that a low dose of haloperidol is used to try to settle Harry during his hospital stays. The registrar is not trying to be unkind by considering the prescription of psychotropic medications. Many factors impact on him: he may have restricted time, or perhaps nurses are pressurising him to 'do something' to alleviate the distress they are witnessing. Harry's family may also express concern at his behaviour. It is more time-consuming and emotionally demanding to engage with the underlying source of distress as well as to try to work out the most appropriate management strategy. It may be that for Harry a rapid discharge back to a familiar environment is in his best interests. Does he still require intravenous antibiotics? Or could he be managed with oral medication in the nursing home setting?

With every pharmaceutical treatment option, it may be helpful to consider the following checklist:

- Is this treatment going to help with comfort (either emotional or physical)?

- What are the consequences (e.g. side effects, renal function) of administering this treatment?

- Is there a non-pharmacological alternative?

- Consider what you would want, in this situation.

---

1    See www.alzheimers.org.uk/thisisme

## 'BEING WITH' RATHER THAN 'DOING FOR'

When you are 'being with' a person dying with dementia:

- You may not be able to respond to cues or draw any conclusions.

- You may not get any verbal or non-verbal communication at all.

Many health professionals would find the above stark truths challenging, and indeed it has been argued that the lack of reciprocity may be a reason for poor dementia care. Nurses have been observed to engage more with patients with whom they can have dialogue (Harrison Dening *et al.* 2012). A study of people with schizophrenia identified that nurses find patients who reject their attempts to care for them challenging (Lorem 2005). Although this research related to patients with schizophrenia, one might reasonably assume that a similar situation may exist in relation to people with advanced dementia. Humans exist in relation to one another, and meaning within relationships is derived from the mutual process of verbal and non-verbal communication.

How can we improve the quality of this aspect of communication, acknowledging the unique challenges described above?

The answer lies in the title of this section – 'being with' rather than 'doing for'.

## SIMPLE THINGS

The issues that cause the most distress to the families of people with dementia are seldom complex. Research has shown that attention to simple human interventions makes a significant difference to how positively families viewed their relative's death. Dignity-promoting activities, such as attending to personal hygiene and mouth care, were among the interventions most highly valued among patients' families (Lawrence *et al.* 2011).

## AFTER DEATH

The preservation of a person's dignity is as important after they have died as before. It is important that the body is gently washed and appropriately dressed, and that bed linen is replaced. Families will have significantly improved memories of this difficult time if respect and care for their loved one is communicated in this way. They may have particular religious requirements relating to who washes or touches the body after death, or how the body is handled. In the case of both Jewish and Muslim families, the faith requires that burial take place as rapidly as possible, ideally within 48 hours. Therefore contacting the relevant services promptly is essential. Out of hours this may still be possible – dedicated religious funeral directors often have a 24-hour telephone line.

### Key points

- This chapter has explored some of the ways in which patients with dementia may receive inadequate or inappropriate emotional care at the end of life.
- Some of the non-physical needs of people dying with dementia have been discussed, and some interventions suggested that may improve the quality of life of the person in this regard.
- It has also been identified that it is both possible and essential for health and social care professionals to acknowledge the personhood and uniqueness of the dying person with dementia, right up until the last moment of their life.

Chapter 4

# Supporting Families through Advanced Dementia and End of Life

**Learning outcomes**

By the end of this chapter you will have:

- Identified the causes of stress commonly experienced by family carers of people with advanced dementia, and considered how these may affect their reactions to loss and grief.

- Suggested ways to minimise the effect of stress on carers.

- Recognised the potential attributes to the caregiving role, and how carers can be supported to gain a positive experience.

- Discussed the decision-making dilemmas experienced by family carers of people with advanced dementia.

- Considered the ethical and legal context of decision-making.

A family carer is someone who gives a substantial amount of unpaid care and support regularly to a relative, partner or friend (Alzheimer's Society 2012). They provide physical, emotional and social support for people with long-term health conditions. It is a challenging role, which most people are unprepared for, and it has physical, psychological, social and financial consequences. Family carers, however, also report positive attributes to caring which include a sense of giving something back to the person they are caring for, becoming closer to them and discovering personal strengths (Peacock *et al.* 2009).

Dementia, like other long-term conditions, takes a protracted and unpredictable course. It has been shown that people with dementia have significant healthcare needs at the end of life comparable to those of cancer patients, and that they are likely to experience these for longer (McCarthy, Addington-Hall and Altmann 1997). Furthermore, recent evidence reports that there is a need to understand more the caregivers' needs related to the management of older people with dementia, as well as the caregivers' own personal needs (McCabe, You and Tatangelo 2016).

The loss of cognitive function in people with end-stage dementia adds additional stress for carers. They can no longer draw on the companionship of their loved one and their partnership in decision-making, particularly the sensitive decisions that need to be made about their end of life care. Levels of psychological stress are significantly higher, and levels of self-efficacy, subjective wellbeing and physical health significantly lower, in dementia carers compared to carers of older people who do not have dementia (Brodaty and Donkin 2009).

There are an estimated 670,000 family carers in the UK for people with dementia, and their contribution saves the UK taxpayer over £8 billion a year (Alzheimer's Society 2012). Providing support to families is integral to the palliative care philosophy and has more recently been recognised as a government priority through the carers strategy (DH 2008b). Its long-term aims are the following:

- Carers will be respected as expert care partners and will have access to the integrated and personalised services they need to support them in their caring role.

- Carers will be able to have a life of their own alongside their caring role.

- Carers will be supported so that they are not forced into financial hardship by their caring role.

- Carers will be supported to stay mentally and physically well and treated with dignity.

Helping carers develop the knowledge, skills and understanding they need to make decisions and care effectively for people at the end of life is part of the *End of Life Care Strategy* (DH 2008a). This chapter focuses on appropriate and timely ways to support professional carers of people with dementia to improve the end of life experience of those with dementia and their family carers.

---

## Key concept

*Stressor:* A state of mental or emotional strain or tension resulting from adverse or demanding circumstances (Oxford English Dictionary).

---

## FAMILY CARERS

Family carers provide 80 per cent of care for older people in the UK (Nolan and Ryan 2011). The majority of family carers of people with dementia are spouses, followed by adult children and children-in-law. The family carer is typically female, although men are beginning to take on the role more frequently. In the United States the number of male family carers increased from 21 per cent in 1996 to 40 per cent in 2008 (Brodaty and Donkin 2009), while in the UK men over 75 are more likely than women to be caring for their spouse (ONS 2005).

The relationship to the person with dementia will influence the type of stressor the family carer experiences. Spouse carers tend to regard caring as an extension of their marital relationship. As the relationship of reciprocity develops into one of dependency, they take on the caring role (Hennings, Froggatt and Payne 2013). Adult children are more likely to face a balancing act between caregiving and the demands of other relationship, family and job commitments. They may have a number of elderly relatives to care for as well as possibly supporting children and grandchildren (Brodaty and Donkin 2009). Adult children will often share the caregiving responsibilities while the spousal caregiver is less likely to have support from others. They are more likely to provide care for their partner with advanced dementia for longer before accepting formal care provision. This is despite the fact that the majority will be elderly with their own healthcare needs (Smale and Dupuis 2004).

## STRESSORS ASSOCIATED WITH CARING FOR SOMEONE WITH DEMENTIA AT THE END OF LIFE

Folkman *et al.* (1986) developed the cognitive theory of psychological stress and coping. Stress is conceptualised as a relationship between the person and the environment that is appraised by the person as challenging their resources and endangering their wellbeing. Coping refers to the person's cognitive and behavioural efforts to reduce, master or tolerate the internal and external demands of the person–environment transaction. Pearlin *et al.* (1990) related this model to carer stress and coping. Carer stress is influenced by the socioeconomic characteristics and skills and resources of the carer as well as the primary and secondary stressors to which they are exposed. Primary stressors are challenges anchored directly in caregiving. Secondary stressors are related to the way the primary stressors interfere with the carer's role and activities outside of caregiving.

Primary dementia caregiving stressors include:

- changes in the cognitive abilities of the person with dementia

- behavioural and emotional changes in the person with dementia

- changes in the relationship between the carer and the person with dementia

- changes in the functional abilities of the person with dementia.

Secondary dementia caregiving stressors include:

- the impact of caring on the carers' usual activities such as work, leisure and looking after themselves, including their own healthcare needs

- conflict or strain in family relationships and friendships

- economic strains

- the need to make decisions on behalf of the person being cared for

- intrapsychic strains such as loss of identity and guilt.

(Oyebode 2008; Zarit and Zarit 2008)

The physical and mental health of carers can suffer directly due to these primary and secondary stressors. Health consequences include physical fatigue and exhaustion or mental health symptoms such as depression and anxiety. Chronic stress affects the body's hormonal and immune systems, leaving carers more vulnerable to disease and infections. The effects of these can be exacerbated as carers may feel unable to take time to attend to their own physical health and emotional needs. They are also more likely to adopt maladaptive health behaviours such as smoking, drinking, a poor diet and lack of exercise (Brodaty and Donkin 2009).

In advanced dementia, stressors surface around the end of life decisions that carers need to make on behalf of their relative. These include choosing the location for receiving end of life care and deciding how to respond to medical crises that will arise (Zarit and Zarit 2008).

## Case study: Carers' thoughts

It's a funny thing caring, you just never feel as though you are doing enough. (Ingvorsen 2013)

The thing is that I always feel guilty: If I am not paying her enough attention, I feel guilty. If I chat and don't get the things done that I need to do to support her, I feel guilty. If I occasionally lose it and feel angry, or fed up with the situation, I feel guilty. It's a lose-lose situation. (Ingvorsen 2013)

Guilt over not doing enough. Guilt over not being there enough. Guilt over wrong choices, broken promises, lost tempers, unfinished conversations. (Gibbons 2012)

I still feel guilt over remembering my Mom ask me, 'Can't I come live with you?', and having to say, 'No.' (Gibbons 2012)

In providing the physical and emotional support for their loved one, some carers find that they adapt to the demands of the role, develop new skills and enhance their coping strategies. For others the years of strain and exhaustion of caregiving may leave them depleted of their personal resources and resilience (Brodaty and Donkin 2009). This highlights the importance of health and social care professionals identifying and offering appropriate support from as early as possible to help carers adapt to the changing demands, and improving their experience in the end of life phase.

## LOSS, GRIEF AND BEREAVEMENT

Stroebe, Stroebe and Hansson (1993) define bereavement as a state of loss, triggering a grief reaction. There are many theories of loss and grief that have common themes to describe the emotions that are considered normal to the grieving process (Bowlby 1980; Kübler-Ross 1969; Parkes 1976; Worden 1991). These include:

- shock, numbness, disbelief

- distress and anger

- depression and despair

- acceptance and resolution.

It is generally accepted that people who have experienced a significant loss will go through some or all of these stages before they reach the point of accepting the loss.

Loss and grief are traditionally associated with the death of a loved one, but for people with protracted illnesses such as dementia, many losses are experienced well before the person dies, and thus loss and grief and the associated emotional responses are an integral part of family carers' lives. A spouse is likely to feel the loss of companionship, affection and intimacy in their relationship with the person with dementia as well as the loss of shared responsibilities and the future they planned together. Adult children may experience loss of support, advice, affection and assistance, or loss of the family kin-keeper bringing everyone together (Zarit and Zarit 2008).

## Loss and guilt

In the later stages of dementia it is often necessary for family carers to seek services and formal support, either in their own home or by admitting their relative into a care home. Although these can remove some of the primary stressors of providing the care, feelings of loss and guilt can arise at relinquishing their caring role (Shanley *et al.* 2011). Spouses can find themselves having to come to terms with living in the wider world without their partner. They live in a period of limbo that can last for months or years. Wishing for this time to end is not uncommon, but these thoughts can fill carers with guilt, knowing it will only end when their partner dies (Hennings *et al.* 2013).

## Anticipatory grief

People may experience grief in anticipation of the death of their loved one. Anticipatory grief and the acknowledgement of the various losses experienced during the course of dementia can lessen the impact of grief after bereavement (Collins *et al.* 1993; Owen, Goode and Haley 2001). There are some barriers to anticipatory grief, however, which include the following:

- An exhaustive routine of providing personal cares that makes it hard to disinvest emotions.

- The impaired cognition of people with advanced dementia means that carers are unable to say the important things they would like to say to their loved one.

(Oyebode 2008)

## Complicated grief

Complicated grief in bereavement may occur when the person is unable to move forward through the grieving process to the point of resolution. Complicated grief may be experienced in several ways:

- chronic grief, of excessive duration

- exaggerated grief, when the person becomes overwhelmed and develops symptoms of severe depression

- delayed grief, when normal grief is inhibited but returns with greater intensity at a future loss.

(Walsh 2011)

The general incidence of complicated grief is unclear. Studies suggest that between 5 per cent and a third of bereaved people show little adaptation to loss after the first year (Payne, Horn and Relf 1999). It is suggested that dementia caregivers are at no greater risk of developing complicated grief than other carers, but certain risk factors have been identified.

Dementia carers may be more vulnerable to complicated grief in bereavement if:

- they do not acknowledge or express grief in response to ongoing losses during dementia caregiving

- they become exhausted or depressed during caregiving

- they lack social support during caregiving

- they are dissatisfied with the professional or nursing home care received by their relative with dementia

- they had an ambivalent relationship with the person they cared for, and are unable to access positive memories.

(Oyebode 2008)

## SUPPORTING FAMILY CARERS THROUGH GRIEF AND LOSS DURING CAREGIVING AND IN BEREAVEMENT

Despite the stressors experienced in caregiving, up to 90 per cent of family carers of people with dementia also report positive experiences. Furthermore, there is evidence that the process of carers reclaiming themselves is significant to the bereavement journey (Peacock *et al.* 2016). Motivation may be fostered by enhancing carers' strengths. Healthcare professionals can help carers develop their coping strategies by targeting social and practical support and resources, and providing information and education that underpins their role as carers (Peacock *et al.* 2009).

If the carer has had a positive relationship with the person with dementia, they may feel a great sense of loss as their loved one's condition deteriorates, but also a strong commitment to providing the needed care. Healthcare professionals can help carers see their caring role as an extension of the love and obligation they feel for the person with dementia (Zarit and Zarit 2008). The carer may feel a sense of failure if the demands of caring become too great and formal care is sought. These feelings are often transferred on to the formal care staff, with the carer showing heightened vigilance over their care (Grande and Keady 2011). Healthcare staff need to respect the role of the carer and involve them in all decisions about the care of their loved one. They could also provide opportunities for the carer to be involved in aspects of caregiving so that they can experience a meaningful and continued commitment (Shanley *et al.* 2011).

Carers can feel very alone; family and friends may withdraw from them, or they may feel too physically and emotionally exhausted to socialise. Healthcare professionals can include an assessment of their family and personal support networks, and encourage them to maintain these contacts. Carers could also be encouraged to enlist the support of respite care services or family and friends so that they regularly have time for themselves (Shanley *et al.* 2011).

Some carers may have had a relationship of conflict with the person with dementia, leaving them feeling ambivalent. They may have a sense of obligation but be resentful or angry about the situation. Non-judgemental conversations about their relationship and their goals in providing care could help them structure their commitment to a level they find acceptable (Zarit and Zarit 2008).

Carers benefit from empathetic understanding as they can often feel judged by family, friends, or society, who are unlikely to understand the full implications of their situation. This support may be found through a friend or a healthcare professional, or through religious and charitable organisations that run carer support groups (Shanley *et al.* 2011).

When the person with dementia dies, the carer may feel the benefit of release from the stressors of caregiving. They may also experience the loss of their investment in caregiving and feel devoid of purpose. Some may feel guilty, perceiving their care to have been less than perfect. At this time it could be helpful for carers to talk to a healthcare professional who knew their relative and the circumstance of their death. It would allow them to ask questions and dispel misconceptions (Oyebode 2008).

A recent model, the Senses Framework, directly addresses family carers' needs and is relationship-centred (Nolan *et al.* 2004). It believes that all parties involved in caring – the cared for, family carers and formal carers – should experience relationships that promote a sense of security, continuity, belonging, purpose, achievement and significance. It identifies key areas to be addressed when providing support to family carers.

- Security:
  - To feel confident in knowledge and ability to provide good care.
  - To have adequate support networks and timely help when required.
  - To be able to relinquish care when appropriate.
- Continuity:
  - To maintain shared pleasures with the cared for.
  - To provide competent standards of care delivered by self or by others.
  - To maintain involvement in care across care environments as desired or appropriate.
- Belonging:
  - To be able to maintain and improve valued relationships.
  - To be able to confide in trusted individuals.
- Purpose:
  - To maintain the dignity, integrity and wellbeing of the cared for.
  - To pursue reciprocal care.
- Achievement:
  - To feel that they have provided the best possible care.
  - To develop new skills and abilities.

- Significance:
  - To feel that their caring is valued and appreciated.

## PARTNERSHIP WORKING WITH FAMILY CARERS AS EXPERTS

It is recognised that a key element to supporting family carers is for healthcare professionals to work in partnership with them. In this model both groups are seen to have differing but complementary forms of expertise. The professional has the knowledge of specific diseases and their treatments, while the family carer has the understanding of the person they care for and what it is like to live with the disease. PREP is a model for working in partnership (Nolan and Ryan 2011):

- **PR**eparedness: Healthcare professionals prepare family carers for their role by providing them with information, advice and skills.

- **E**nrichment: Healthcare professionals work actively with family carers and the cared for person in order to enrich their experience and improve their relationships.

- **P**redictability: Healthcare professionals try and make the future as predictable as possible so that carers can prepare for the eventualities.

Involving family carers has been shown to contribute to improvements in care, and is seen as a high priority by people with dementia, carers and professionals (RCN 2011).

## SUPPORTING FAMILY CARERS TO STAY CONNECTED WITH THEIR RELATIVE

Communication is an essential part of person-centred care. As dementia progresses, the person with dementia and their carer have to adapt to changes that occur in their communication partnership – they need to place greater reliance on non-verbal communication. A failure to adapt could lead to feelings of alienation for the carer (Allan and Killick 2008). Encouraging the carer to engage in relaxation activities with the person with dementia such as gentle hand massage and listening to their favourite music together could help them remain connected, even when verbal communication is no longer possible (Ghiotti 2009).

Enhancing the quality of relationships and the rewards of caring are key components of the PREP model. The feelings of guilt and sadness can be lessened for carers who experience a sense of satisfaction with their caregiving (Nolan and Ryan 2011).

## SUPPORTING FAMILY CARERS IN END OF LIFE DECISION-MAKING

End of life decisions may range from the need for the carers to take over tasks such as washing, dressing and feeding to placement of their relative in a care home and issues around their medical treatments (Baldwin 2008). Chapter 1 looked at some of the practical approaches and the ethical frameworks around end of life decision-making. It referred to advance care planning as a nuanced and sensitive way of initiating discussions and decisions about end of life care. It is important for the main healthcare provider to begin advance care planning with the person with dementia and their family as soon as possible, and to involve the person with dementia for as long as possible, as those who lose capacity to make complex decisions can continue to express their feelings and emotions for some more time (Mental Capacity Act 2005).

In advanced stages people with dementia are not always able to participate in meaningful discussions. Carers become proxy decision-makers and often feel unprepared for this role. Recent evidence reports the possibility that family carers have a low-to-moderate agreement with a person with dementia on preferences for end of life treatment (Harrison Dening et al. 2016), emphasising the need to ascertain views early in the disease before their ability to consider the future is compromised (Harrison Dening, Jones and Sampson 2013).

Treatment decisions related to nutrition and hydration, cardiopulmonary resuscitation, transfers to acute care setting and use of antibiotic therapy can be stressful, particularly if a crisis occurs and there have been no prior discussions. Family carers do not usually feel competent in making such decisions, and although they want their relative to die with comfort and dignity, to waiver treatment can make them feel like they are abandoning them (Caron, Griffith and Arcand 2005; Forbes *et al.* 2000).

The Mental Capacity Act (2005) states that decisions about the care of people with advanced dementia should be through consensus among healthcare professionals and family carers, with consideration of the patient's known or perceived wishes, beliefs and values. Any decision made should be in the best interests of the person with dementia. A recent and updated guide to Do Not Attempt Cardiopulmonary Resuscitation (DNACPR) by the Resuscitation Council UK (2016) includes more details for decision-making for those without capacity.

Reaching consensus about treatment decisions can be difficult. Different cultures and religions have different views about death and dying. Some strive to preserve life regardless of the cost of suffering, while others value the quality of end of life. Conflict can arise among family members as people may have different values and interpretations of their culture and the perceived wishes of the person with dementia. In some cultures, for example, it would be seen in a negative way to ask for and accept formal care. The community may judge the extended family poorly if the children did not fulfil their obligations of providing all the care (Connolly, Sampson and Purandare 2012).

Empathic rapport with an emphasis on working in partnership could help healthcare professionals to build trust with the families and communities. To promote empathy, healthcare professionals need to have an awareness of their own values towards death and dying and to understand how it may be different to those they are caring for (Caron *et al.* 2005). Ongoing communication with the healthcare team can improve carers' understanding of the dementia trajectory and provide information on the burdens and benefits of medical treatments (Caron *et al.* 2005). This will help them make informed decisions.

## Case study: Family decision-making

Badriya moved to the UK in the 1980s to marry Hafeez. They have two daughters – Seeta is married and has a child with cerebral palsy, and Rashida is studying at the local university. Hafeez is self-employed and works long hours. Badriya has numerous medical problems, including vascular dementia and heart failure. She has a leg ulcer which is proving difficult to heal, partly because of her poor circulation and oedema, and partly because she is inclined to try to remove dressings that the nurses apply. The district nurse suggests to Hafeez that they consider admission to a nursing home, but Hafeez becomes angry and offended. He tells the nurse that his daughters will care for her when she needs it. He accuses the nurse of using wound dressings that are uncomfortable, and suggests that this is the reason for Badriya's current unsettled state. The nurse believes that Badriya is approaching end of life and needs greater care input, but is worried about causing offence by discussing it again.

- It is possible that district nursing staff visiting to attend to Badriya's wound have been influenced by a perception that she has a large and supportive family and have therefore not been particularly proactive in acknowledging the difficulties that Badriya's family are experiencing trying to keep her safe and at home.

- Although Hafeez believes that home is the right place for her to be despite increasingly complex care requirements, it is possible that there will be some family tension with regards to how to facilitate this care arrangement.

- Badriya may have been a big support for Seeta caring for her child with cerebral palsy. Now Seeta has the further strain of caring for her mother as well.

- Rashida may feel some regrets if she falls behind with her studies because of the demands of caring, as well as missing out on university social life.

It may be that the nurses need to listen carefully to each family member's concerns as a group, and to highlight in a non-judgemental way the tensions that exist. A compromise may be possible – for example, could a sitter be obtained for part of the time? Could an occasional respite admission help? Are there any members of the community available and willing to help? What are the issues relating to the wound dressing – does Hafeez understand the reasons for his wife's wound not healing or is he blaming the treatment? Careful explanation and empathy could help. A case review meeting could involve the general practitioner (GP) as well as the district nursing team and the family.

In situations where values are not shared, difficult conflicts can arise between healthcare professionals and families or between family members, resulting in negative emotions for families such as guilt, fear and anger. These will impact on their grieving process. It is important to try to resolve any conflicting opinions, and case review meetings are advocated (Zarit and Zarit 2008). Anyone involved in the care of the person with dementia should meet together with the healthcare professionals. This way everyone receives the same information at the same time, views can be aired, and the benefits and burdens of different scenarios discussed with everyone.

## SAFEGUARDING ISSUES

People with dementia who have lost their decision-making capacity are vulnerable to care decisions being made that are not in their best interests. Such decisions may be made with malicious or non-malicious intent. Consider the following: a husband is determined to honour his marriage vows and continue to care for his wife with dementia. Without support or respite care, tensions build between them. His wife does not seem to recognise him most of the time and pushes him away when he tries to do anything for her. She is incontinent and unable to maintain her own personal hygiene. In his frustration he starts to shout at her regularly and uses physical force to get her to comply with him. Ideally healthcare professionals will pick up this situation, and with empathetic understanding and discussion, the husband may be encouraged to accept formal care for his wife. If he does not and the situation continues, the healthcare professionals can refer to the independent mental capacity advocate (IMCA), who will represent the person with dementia in the decision-making process. Essentially they make sure that the Mental Capacity Act 2005 is being followed. If they have concerns, they can refer the case to the Court of Protection. The Court of Protection has the power to make a declaration as to the lawfulness or otherwise of any specific act relating to a patient's care or treatment (Mental Capacity Act 2005).

## Case study: Ethical dilemmas

Harriet has been having increasing difficulty swallowing her food, despite a consultation with a speech and language therapist and an individualised care plan specifying the appropriate texture for her food. The staff's fear that she may be aspirating on her fluids and diet is confirmed when she develops a high temperature and productive cough. She is having difficulty swallowing even liquid oral antibiotics, and after some discussion with her family and the GP she is admitted to hospital for intravenous (IV) antibiotic therapy. The family is informed that her prognosis appears grave, and discussions are had about transferring her back to the nursing home to allow a natural death. The family is upset at how quickly this decision has been made, and resist this strongly. They request that she is given a full 24 hours of IV antibiotics. The following morning she appears more alert and manages some sips of tea, although her swallow remains poor.

As Harriet continues to improve on the antibiotics, her family is placed in a difficult position. She is clearly very frail, and the occurrence of a chest infection makes it highly likely that a similar problem will arise in the near future. Will Harriet be admitted to hospital for IV antibiotics each time she gets a chest infection, or should she be kept comfortable in the care home on the next occurrence? Should she undergo an operation, with the associated risks, to have a PEG (percutaneous gastrostomy) tube inserted to maintain her nutritionally? Not only do they not know the precise outcome of any decision they will make, they are also unable to involve Harriet in these discussions.

In the absence of any Advance Statement, the ethical principles of beneficence and non-maleficence are predominant. In this situation a balance of evidence- and values-based medicine is needed in the decision-making process (NICE 2010). The decision-makers need to know the evidence-based facts about the dementia disease trajectory and any proposed treatments. It is outlined in Chapter 2 that in the terminal stages of dementia active treatments for physical illness and functional decline, including administering antibiotics and the insertion of a PEG, do not necessarily prolong life, as they do not limit the progression of the dementia (Hurley *et al.* 1996; Meier *et al.* 2001; Mitchell *et al.* 2004). However, as discussed in Chapter 1, determining the end stage of dementia is problematic, and therefore decisions about care should not be based on survival alone. The values-based medicine takes account of the burdens and benefits of various treatments, the person's quality of life, their degree of suffering and their known or perceived wishes and values. In this situation the family needs to consider what Harriet's values and wishes might be. They may be able to think back to a time when someone close to her was dying, and what her thoughts were then. They also need to consider the level of distress that Harriet experienced with her admission to hospital and the invasive procedure of putting in a cannula for IV antibiotics. Will recurrent admissions to hospital reduce the quality of her end of life, and is the family prepared that she may die in hospital on one of these occasions?

There are frequent situations in end of life decision-making for people with advanced dementia when it would seem that the ethical principle of autonomy conflicts with those of beneficence and non-maleficence.

Take the case of Alfred who has advanced dementia. His family says that after he was diagnosed with dementia he told them that he did not want to go into hospital or a care home, and he did not want any treatment that would prolong his life. He did not make a formal Advance Decision to Refuse Treatment (ADRT). Consider the following scenarios and what would influence the decisions that need to be made about Alfred's care and treatment.

## Case study: Best interests

- In the advanced stages of dementia Alfred appears quite content and shows pleasure by smiling when his family visit. He eats little but seems to still enjoy some of his favourite foods that are easy to swallow. He gets a chest infection that could potentially be cured with oral antibiotics. It does not distress him to take the antibiotic in liquid form.

- Alfred falls and fractures his femur. The best way to manage his pain is through an operation to stabilise the fracture.

- Alfred's wife Brenda, his main carer, becomes too unwell to continue to care for him. He is unsafe to be left on his own, even for short periods of time.

Should you respect Alfred's autonomy by complying with his previous known wishes?

In bioethics, autonomy is the dominant ethical principle based on the individual and their right to make choices (Beauchamp and Childress 2001). Kitwood (1997, p.8) argues that personhood does not depend on ability or capacity, but is '…a standing or status that is bestowed upon one human being by others, in the context of relationship and social being. It implies recognition, respect and trust.' Baldwin (2008) suggests that for people who lack capacity to make rational decisions, personhood should be at the centre of ethical reasoning.

Decisions may be made for Alfred that go against his earlier wishes but that are more likely to uphold his personhood. In the third scenario the decision may be that Alfred needs to go into a care home. By trying to keep him at home he may be in danger of harm and his wife will likely continue with poor health trying to cope. This will be detrimental to his relationship with his family and therefore his personhood. The family can further uphold his personhood by ensuring he has items that are familiar to him in his room in the care home, they visit regularly and tell his life story to the staff, and his wife takes on acts of caring, as she is able.

Hope (2009) suggests that both the past wishes and feelings of the person and their current wishes and feelings should be taken into consideration, although they may be quite different. In the first scenario, taking the antibiotic medication may return Alfred to his previous quality of life before the infection where he showed moments of pleasure and was not unduly distressed. These current emotions are different to the horror and distress he experienced at diagnosis. A different set of considerations would need to be discussed if he required hospital admission for IV antibiotics.

Without admission to hospital in the second scenario, pain control would be difficult and could seriously affect Alfred's quality of end of life. The healthcare professionals and family could look to uphold his personhood by coordinating post-operative care in the community, making his stay in hospital as short as possible. They could also provide the hospital staff with information about him so they can give individualised care. The 'This is me' leaflet,[1] discussed in Chapters 1 and 2, is a useful tool.

A best interests decision is made within the legal framework of the Mental Capacity Act 2005, for those who lack the capacity to make the decision. The Deprivation of Liberty Safeguards (DOLS, DH 2009a) are part of the Mental Capacity Act. They aim to make sure that people who require care in care homes, hospitals and supported living are looked after in a way that does not inappropriately restrict their freedom. If staff within these organisations feel that in order to maintain a person's safety it is necessary to have control of their care or movements over a prolonged period of time, a DOLS will need to be obtained. The safeguards are designed to ensure that a person's loss of liberty is lawful and that the person is protected. The organisation will need to show that the person is being cared for in the least restrictive manner. This, in essence, corresponds to ensuring all efforts are made to uphold their personhood.

---

1    See www.alzheimers.org.uk/thisisme

## Key points

- Family carers are diverse in age and circumstances, and there are many factors that will influence their experience of caring. These include socioeconomic factors, their personality and coping strategies, and their relationship with the person they care for.

- Health and social care professionals need to recognise the primary and secondary stressors of caregiving, and address the carers' needs with respect to these.

- Health and social care professionals need to work in partnership with the carer, supporting them to stay connected to their relative, and to make informed decisions on their behalf within a legal and ethical context.

- Health and social care professionals need to provide carers with knowledge and support, and develop a trusting relationship at an early stage. This will help carers build on their strengths, develop skills and adjust to the changing demands of caregiving. This, in turn, should help them achieve greater psychological and physical resilience when faced with the end of life period of their loved one and in bereavement.

- A minority of dementia carers will experience complicated grief in bereavement. Understanding the risk factors for complicated grief in dementia carers can help health and social care professionals identify those who are vulnerable, and put appropriate support mechanisms in place pre- and post-bereavement.

Chapter 5

# Supporting the Health and Social Care Workforce to Provide End of Life Care for People with Dementia

**Learning outcomes**

At the end of this chapter, you will:

- Recognise the context in which the dementia and end of life care workforce is developing, and the challenges faced when providing end of life care for people with dementia.
- Understand the education, training and development needs of the workforce, and the influence of these on the quality of their work life and delivery of care.
- Identify how to empower professionals in health and social care to deliver end of life care for people with dementia care through:
  - education, training and practice development
  - effective leadership and teamworking.
- Be able to acknowledge the individual support needs of staff.

End of life care for people with dementia has become a healthcare priority (Watson, Hockley and Murray 2010). It poses particular challenges to those providing services because of a lack of confidence in their skills, a sense of helplessness and a need for improved knowledge about dementia and palliative care (Chang *et al.* 2009). In common with people with cancer, those with dementia may experience multiple and complex problems with symptoms such as pain, swallowing difficulties, repeated infections, urinary incontinence, constipation and poor nutrition at the end of life. However, people with dementia and their families may experience these symptoms for longer periods of time compared to those with advanced cancer, and are less able to communicate the effects of these symptoms or their distress (Mitchell *et al.* 2009).

In addition, the prolonged and unpredictable dying trajectory associated with dementia impacts on the place of death – people with dementia are most likely to die in their own homes, care homes and acute hospitals, with few dying in hospices or accessing specialist palliative care (NEoLCP 2010). The prolonged dying trajectory, coupled with differing philosophies and approaches to care across care settings, can present challenges to the transferability and delivery of the palliative and end of life care developed within hospices (Rowlands and Rowlands 2012). Individual and organisational learning and support are therefore required to develop innovative practice, service models and frameworks of care that are appropriate for people with dementia at the end of life.

The previous chapters in this book have demonstrated some of the challenges faced and the skills, knowledge and commitment required by family members, professionals and support workers in health and social care to provide high-quality person-centred care for people with dementia at the end of life. Prompted by the *National Dementia Strategy* (DH 2009b) recommendation for 'an informed and effective workforce', education, training and support are widely acknowledged as fundamental to ensuring that the health and social care workforce are able to meet the needs of people with dementia including those at the end of life (Rowlands and Rowlands 2012; van der Steen *et al.* 2013).

The 'workforce' includes any member of staff working in health and social care with people with dementia, ranging from general practitioners (GPs) and hospital consultants to health and social care support workers. It also includes education for commissioners and education providers who aim to ensure the availability and accessibility to training and education at a range of levels to meet service needs. End of life education is necessary for the workforce to be competent and up to date in knowledge and practice (National Palliative and End of Life Care Partnership 2015) as well as in more specific groups such as people with dementia. Palliative care and hospice advocacy groups such as the National Council for Palliative Care (NCPC) and Hospice UK advocate a partnership approach (Hospice UK 2015), in which palliative care services learn from dementia services, and vice versa (NCPC 2009). As education alone is not enough to change practice (Shershneva *et al.* 2010), leaders within services are recognised as being critical to setting an appropriate learning culture and context for the delivery of high-quality care, effective teamworking and support to care staff (APPG 2008).

This chapter explores the impact of education and support on the quality of care, and provides suggestions for empowering the health and social care workforce to be innovative in end of life care for people with dementia.

## EDUCATION AND TRAINING

There are currently 850,000 people living with dementia in the UK, and this number is expected to rise over the coming years (Prince *et al.* 2014). It is predominantly a disease of the elderly, who are more likely to suffer co-morbidities and have a need to access health and social care for a variety of reasons including those associated with their dementia. This means that the majority of those who work in health and social care will have significant contact with people with dementia. This constitutes a large workforce that requires education to be confident and competent in how they can support people (and their families) with dementia at the end of their lives.

There have been a variety of examples of a systematic approach to the education of the workforce. For example, Health Education England (DH 2015), responsible for overseeing education and training within the health and care system, developed a three-tier programme of training to be rolled out nationally:

| | |
|---|---|
| **Tier 1** | Awareness-raising, in terms of knowledge, skills and attitudes, for all those working in health and care. |
| **Tier 2** | Knowledge, skills and attitudes for roles that have regular contact with people living with dementia. |
| **Tier 3** | Enhancing the knowledge, skills and attitudes for key staff (experts) working with people living with dementia, designed to support them in leadership roles. |

A white paper defining optimal palliative care in older people with dementia (see van der Steen *et al.* 2013) recommended that all health staff should be competent in a range of domains (e.g. person-centred care, psychological and social care, advance care planning, symptom control, family care, prognostication, futile treatments, etc.). The European Association of Palliative Care (EAPC) (see Gamondi, Larkin and Payne 2013a, 2013b) and the *End of Life Care Strategy* (DH 2008a) have also developed a three-tier framework to deliver education to healthcare professionals by mapping competences to the degree of palliative care involvement that an individual has in their everyday practice.

**Table 5.1 Workforce groups and levels
of skill, knowledge and education**

| Group definition (DH 2008a) | Minimum skill and knowledge level (DH 2008a) | EAPC-agreed levels of education for professionals involved in palliative care (Gamondi *et al.* 2013a) |
| --- | --- | --- |
| *Group A:* Specialist palliative care staff; work entirely focused on people at the end of their lives. | Highest levels, through specialist training. To include all of the common core competences. | *Specialist palliative care:* Provided in services whose main activity is delivery of palliative care. Care for patients with complex and difficult needs. Requires higher level of education, staff and resources. Usually taught at postgraduate level and reinforced through continuing professional development (CPD). |
| *Group B:* Staff who frequently deal with end of life care as part of their role. | Staff need to be enabled to develop or apply existing skills and knowledge to the principles and competences. May require additional specialist training. | *General palliative care:* Provided by primary care professionals and specialists treating patients with life-threatening diseases who have good basic palliative care skills and knowledge. Should be available to professionals involved more frequently in palliative care but who do not provide palliative care as the main focus of their work. Depending on discipline, may be taught at undergraduate or postgraduate level or through CPD. |

| Group C: Staff working within other services who are involved with end of life care infrequently. | Good basic grounding in the principles and competences alongside knowledge of where to seek expert advice or where to refer on to. | *Palliative care approach:* A way to integrate palliative care methods and procedures in settings not specialised in palliative care. Should be made available to GPs and staff in general hospitals, as well as nursing services and care homes. May be taught through undergraduate learning or through CPD. |
|---|---|---|

*Source: Adapted from DH (2008a) and Gamondi (2013a)*

Furthermore, in the UK, a range of policy reports and documents such as the National Institute for Health and Care Excellence's (NICE) *Quality Standards for Dementia* (2016), The Choice in End of Life Care Programme Board's *What's Important to Me* (2015) and *The Government Response to the Review of Choice in End of Life Care* (NHS Finance and Operations/ NHS Group/NHS Clinical Services 2016) all advocate the need for education to enable a competent workforce providing end of life care.

Bringing the HEE programme and the EAPC/Department of Health (DH) frameworks together will help to determine the level of palliative and dementia care training required by individual staff, depending on their roles, to provide optimal palliative and end of life care for people with dementia. It is clear that ongoing collaboration and conversations between specialists in palliative and dementia care will enable services and knowledge to be developed together, enabling better and best care for people with dementia and their families.

Several policy documents have been produced with the explicit aim of improving the quality of care given to people with dementia and people at the end of life. The table below presents three of these, which demonstrates that there are areas of common principles which can help commissioners and managers to focus on a plan for educational interventions in a variety of clinical settings to provide end of life care for people with dementia.

**Table 5.2 Examples of dementia and palliative care competencies**

| Common Core Principles for Supporting People with Dementia (Skills for Care and Skills for Health and DH 2011) | Common Core Competences and Principles for Health and Social Care Workers Working with Adults at the End of Life (NEoLCP 2009) | EAPC Ten Core Competences in Palliative Care (Gamondi *et al.* 2013a, 2013b) |
|---|---|---|
| 1. Know the early signs of dementia. | 1. The choices and priorities of the individual are at the centre of all end of life care planning and delivery. | 1. Apply core constituents of palliative care in the setting where patients and families are based. |
| 2. Early diagnosis of dementia helps people receive information, support and treatment at the earliest possible stage. | 2. Effective, straightforward, sensitive and open communication between individuals, families, friends and workers underpins all planning and activity. Communication reflects an understanding of the significance of each individual's beliefs and needs. | 2. Enhance physical comfort throughout patients' disease trajectories. |

| | | |
|---|---|---|
| 3. Communicate sensitively to support meaningful interaction. | 3. High-quality end of life care is delivered through close multidisciplinary and interagency working. Through partnership working, the needs of the individual are articulated, shared, understood and reviewed. By developing and utilising networks, the right resources and support are identified and utilised. | 3. Meet patients' psychological needs. |
| 4. Promote independence and encourage activity. | 4. Individuals and their families and friends are well informed about the range of options and resources available to them to enable them to be involved in the planning, developing and evaluating of end of life care plans and services. | 4. Meet patients' social needs. |
| 5. Recognise the signs of distress resulting from confusion, and respond by diffusing a person's anxiety and supporting their understanding of the events they experience. | 5. Care is delivered in a sensitive, person-centred way that takes account of the circumstances, wishes and priorities of the individual and their family and friends. | 5. Meet patients' spiritual needs. |

| | | |
|---|---|---|
| 6. Family members and other carers are valued, respected and supported, just like those they care for, and are helped to gain access to dementia care. | 6. Care and support are available to, and continue for, anyone affected by the end of life, and death, of the individual. | 6. Respond to the needs of the family carers in relation to short-, medium- and long-term patient care goals. |
| 7. Managers need to take responsibility to ensure members of their team are trained and well supported to meet the needs of people with dementia. | 7. Workers are supported to develop knowledge, skills and attitudes that enable them to initiate and deliver high-quality end of life care or, where appropriate, to seek advice and guidance from other colleagues. Workers recognise the importance of their CPD, and take responsibility for it. | 7. Respond to the challenges of clinical and ethical decision-making in palliative care. |
| 8. Work as part of a multi-agency team to support the person with dementia. | 8. Competences: a. Communication skills. b. Assessment and care planning. c. Symptom management, maintaining comfort and wellbeing. d. Advance care planning. e. Overarching values and knowledge. | 8. Practise comprehensive care coordination and interdisciplinary teamwork across all settings where palliative care is offered. |

| |
|---|
| 9. Develop interpersonal and communication skills appropriate to palliative care. |
| 10. Practise self-awareness and undergo CPD. |

It is encouraging that both palliative and dementia care providers are looking at their workforce needs. For example, Hospice UK's (2015, p.37) 'Hospice-enabled dementia care' guide specifically recommends education ranging from awareness to funding for higher level dementia qualifications, and Northern Ireland Hospice now delivers a well-evaluated European Certificate in Holistic Dementia Care.[1]

In the context of delivering palliative care for people with dementia, health and social care professionals require expertise in managing behavioural problems and in anticipating, assessing and managing physical, psychosocial and emotional issues. Communicating with people with dementia and their families also requires special skills because the cognitive problems associated with dementia complicate decision-making around a host of issues. Furthermore, support for families is needed to help them in their role as proxy decision-makers in more advanced dementia, and to deal with a high burden of care and chronic grief caused by the continuing deterioration of their loved one with dementia (van der Steen *et al.* 2013).

Education can improve staff confidence, but there are numerous challenges in provision, such as recognising whose responsibility it is, in a complex health and social care system, to ensure that the carers receive appropriate and

---

1    See www.nihospicecare.com/Certificate_In_Dementia

sustained training. Education is cited as an intervention that can improve dementia end of life care in, for example, care homes, albeit recent reviews by Kupeli *et al.* (2016b) and Goodman *et al.* (2011, 2016) emphasise a wide range of other contextual aspects such as working relationships or financial incentives. It is therefore wise to consider education as one part of an intervention to improve care. However, there is evidence that educational interventions do appear to increase staff knowledge and confidence in end of life care (Spilsbury, Hanratty and McCaughan 2015), and there are a variety of models available – Table 5.3 gives some examples.

**Table 5.3 Examples of education initiatives**

| | |
|---|---|
| ABC End of Life Care Home Education across Bedfordshire, Hertfordshire and Luton (Hospice of St Francis, Peace Hospice Care, Isabel Hospice, Keech Hospice Care) | A programme of flexible face-to-face and e-learning education with clinical mentorship and support (including hospice-based staff), designed to meet the end of life care education needs of trained and untrained staff working across residential and nursing homes and domiciliary agencies. Three formal evaluations, including comparing it to the Gold Standards Framework care home programme (Cook, Cook and Driver 2012; Pyper *et al.* 2013), have shown this to be value for money and to improve care. In 2011–14, 181 homes and 2059 individuals completed the ABC programme. In 2014, 24 homes and 42 staff completed the 'Train the Trainer' programme (Russell 2014b). |
| Six Steps to Success Programme (St John's Hospice, Lancaster) | Workshop-style training programme developed by the Greater Manchester and Cheshire Cancer Network, the Merseyside and Cheshire Cancer Network and the Cumbria and Lancashire End of Life Care Network, with support from the National End of Life Care Programme. It enables care homes to implement the structured organisational change required to deliver the best end of life care. |

| | |
|---|---|
| Six Steps[a] continuous quality improvement programme for care homes, nursing homes and domiciliary agencies (St Luke's Hospice, Plymouth) | Comprises a series of workshops designed to provide care agencies with the toolkit to meet Care Quality Commission (CQC) end of life essential standards, DH end of life and/or dementia and/or learning disability quality markers. Also linked to the Skills for Care's end of life qualification, and has an implementation programme for others to use – 68 organisations and 118 individuals have taken part locally. |
| Gold Standards Framework[b] | A well-known and popular model that offers comprehensive, evidence-based quality improvement training programmes for all generalists delivering care to people nearing the end of their Life. Programmes are mapped to the Skills for Care's end of life qualifications. Programmes have been formally evaluated to show improvement in the quality and quantity of communication and collaboration between nursing home staff and primary care and specialist practitioners (Badger et al. 2012), symptom control and team communication (Hall et al. 2011) and advance care planning (Hockley et al. 2010). There is also evidence of the value of reflective and team debriefing approaches to support (Hockley 2014). |
| PACE (Palliative Care Education) Care Home Support[c] (Norfolk Community Health and Care NHS Trust) | The PACE education team includes care home facilitators whose role is to help care home staff develop their end of life care skills. Working within a wider group, including representatives from Macmillan, Norfolk Hospice, Health Education East of England and the Norfolk & Suffolk Palliative Care Academy, they offer education and service development to care homes throughout Norfolk. More than 80 per cent of care homes with nursing, and nearly half of all 400-plus care homes, have received support from this group. Activities include the Six Steps programme, e-learning and face-to-face training. |

| Three approaches to delivering end-of-life education to care homes in a region of south east England | A comparison of the Six Steps programme, Gold Standards Framework and an action learning project. All demonstrated improvements in end of life care in the care homes (Booth *et al.* 2014). |
|---|---|

[a] See www.stlukes-hospice.org.uk/education-six-steps-programme
[b] See www.goldstandardsframework.org.uk/training-programmes
[c] See www.norfolkcommunityhealthandcare.nhs.uk/s_PACE/Pages/courses/six-steps.htm

Other education interventions include *Local training and development reviews* (Skills for Care and Skills for Health and DH 2011), outlined below, which has been developed to help service managers review the workplace and to plan training and development in relation to caring for people with dementia. It can be used as a benchmarking record to monitor improvements and changes that are introduced to the training and development available for the workforce.

### Table 5.4 Training and development reviews

| |
|---|
| Describe the services you provide for people with dementia |
| Based on the needs of people with dementia who use your service, describe the ambition for the service and for workforce development in your local context |
| Who interacts with the person with dementia?<br>• Which people?<br>• Which teams? |
| What skills do they need?<br>• Indicative behaviours from common core principles<br>• Specialist skills in caring for people with dementia |
| What training and development is currently available? Audit:<br>• Content<br>• Access<br>• Resources<br>• Qualifications<br>• Outcomes – what the person and their family using the service experiences |

What training needs to be accessed, designed and delivered?
- What kind of learning works best for the workforce?
- Negotiate with training providers – are the programmes developed using national occupational standards?
- Use qualifications and credit framework units to ensure the workforce achieves a recognised standard of skills
- Develop your own learning programme – use national occupational standards to inform your context-specific competences

How will the training and development be delivered? Examples:
- Corporate induction
- Local networks
- Regular staff meetings and training sessions
- Appraisals
- Dementia conference for full organisation and partners
- Clinical supervision (group and/or individual)
- Action learning groups
- Others (specify)

*Source: Adapted from Skills for Care and Skills for Health and DH (2011)*

Furthermore, the generic seven common core principles and competences for social care and health workers working with adults at the end of life (Skills for Care and Skills for Health 2014) provide a framework for people engaged in managing, commissioning and delivering end of life care and support.

## DELIVERING EDUCATION

Research finds that new knowledge alone rarely results in sustained changes to practice (Broad 1997). Reviewing the evidence, Cromwell and Kolb (2004) surmise that lasting practice change requires an effective training programme, learner preparation prior to the training, and sustained and targeted support following it. Support and encouragement from supervisors or managers was found to positively influence the workers' confidence and their intent to use new knowledge.

Key components to delivering training and engaging in learning include:

- *Facilitation:* A facilitator's role is to lead the educational experience by shaping and guiding a group in the process of working together to achieve identified goals. The skills required of a facilitator are:

  ○ active listening

  ○ giving and receiving constructive feedback

  ○ asking enabling questions

  ○ challenging and supporting (Titchen, Dewing and Manley 2013).

- *Reflective practice:* The ability to reflect on an action so as to engage in a process of continuous learning (Schön 1983). This is the process of critically analysing and drawing on theory to evaluate existing practice and to generate new knowledge and ideas. There are different frameworks for structuring reflection; Gibbs (1988) has produced a well-known cycle of reflection comprising six stages and a series of cue questions.

## EXPERIENTIAL LEARNING

Kolb (1984, p.38) integrates reflective practice into his model of the 'experiential learning cycle' in which he theorises that 'learning is a process whereby knowledge is created through the transformation of experience'. It is a cyclical model made up of four stages, as illustrated below.

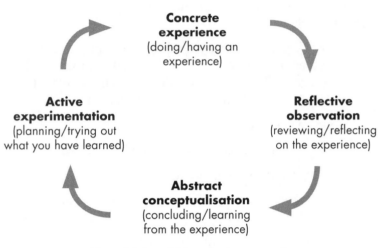

Figure 5.1 A model for reflecting on practice

Through this model Kolb (1984) addresses four different learning styles based on each stage. These styles are:

- *Assimilating:* People learn when presented with sound logic and theories.

- *Converging:* People learn when provided with practical applications of concepts and theories.

- *Accommodating:* People learn when provided with 'hands-on' experience.

- *Diverging:* People learn by observing and collecting a wide range of material.

Although individuals tend to predominantly favour one way of learning, Kolb (1984) suggests that effective learning is achieved when a person progresses through all stages of the cycle, engaging with all four learning styles.

To meet the needs of a vast workforce, several interactive online training resources have been developed in end of life care and in dementia care. These initiatives can be used to complement and support a variety of learning experiences by individuals, small groups or in the classroom. They adopt the principles of experiential learning by providing a mix of audio and video materials, information giving, case studies and participatory exercises. This accommodates for differences in individuals' learning styles and maximises the learning experience through activity, reflection, theory and application (Rogers 2007).

While there remains some ambivalence about e-learning as an education method for busy clinicians (Russell 2016), it has gained popularity (Greenhalgh 2001). One of its advantages is that it can reach great numbers of learners at the same time (Wee 2012), as well as being a flexible and accessible learning method for individuals (Ahmed 2010; Cook *et al.* 2008; Ruggeri, Farrington and Brayne 2013). E-learning has been used in a wide range of ways, from palliative care education in Sub-Saharan Africa (Rawlinson and Luyirika 2014) to blended learning in English care homes (Farrington 2014). A recent study of GPs' end of life educational needs reported that e-learning was the preferred method, with blended approaches recommended (Magee and Koffman 2014).

There are a variety of online resources available that are useful especially in a blended learning or flipped classroom approach. As well as the few examples cited below, there are other examples from NHS trusts and universities that develop their own online dementia education programmes – for example, Barbara's Story, the training programme of Guy's and St Thomas' NHS Foundation Trust.[2] This follows an older woman called Barbara through her healthcare journey as her dementia gradually advances and she receives a diagnosis of terminal cancer. It explores the challenges she faces when she comes into contact with NHS staff at home and in hospital, and highlights the importance of everyone's contribution, from doctor to community nurse, and from support worker to taxi driver, in creating a safe and positive environment.

---

2   See www.guysandstthomas.nhs.uk/education-and-training/staff-training/barbaras-story.aspx

**Table 5.5 Examples of e-learning**

| Source | Comment |
| --- | --- |
| e-ELCA[a] | End of life care peer-reviewed programme with over 150 interactive sessions (including dementia-specific modules), supported by the Association for Palliative Medicine and NHS Health Education England. It can be used as a single learner or by groups. Following the publication of the *Care of Dying Adults in the Last Days of Life* (NICE 2015), e-ELCA sessions have also been highlighted as a resource to help with implementation of the guidelines. |
| Social Care Institute for Excellence[b] | Information, guidance, resources and accredited training for anyone supporting people with dementia. Includes a section on end of life care in dementia. |
| Health Education England (HEE)[c] | Developed e-learning sessions in dementia designed to familiarise health and social care staff with recognising and understanding dementia, and to be able to signpost appropriate support. |
| The National Skills Academy[d] | Incorporates six video dramatisations across different settings. Learners can follow Maggie and Mick as Maggie receives a diagnosis of dementia, gets help at home and moves into a residential care home. They can then follow Marty and Mary, and Marty's family, as he receives emergency medical care, stays on an acute hospital ward and nears the end of his life. |

[a] See www.e-lfh.org.uk/programmes/end-of-life-care
[b] See www.scie.org.uk/dementia/e-learning
[c] See https://hee.nhs.uk/our-work/hospitals-primary-community-care/mental-health-learning-disability/mental-health/dementia
[d] See www.nsahealth.org.uk/e-learning/courses-we-offer/286:stand-by-me-dementia-free-e-learning-course

In addition to the need for education in dementia and palliative care for health and social carers, there have been various models of training developed to address this:

- *Train the Trainer:* Experts give training and skills to a core group of staff within an organisation, to facilitate a specific programme of learning for their colleagues (Connell *et al.* 2002). The programme becomes more sustainable if the core group of staff continue to act as a link between the experts and the organisation, and form a network of champions sharing good practice.

- *Action learning groups:* A team applies the experiential learning cycle to work activities and, through action planning, a continuing cycle of improvement based on evidence and the practicalities of the clinical setting is promoted. The team plans future action within a supportive milieu, requiring regular meetings to share problems and experiences (Manley 2005).

## PRACTICE DEVELOPMENT

Implementing theory into practice frequently requires a change in the culture and practices of an organisation, as well as a systematic approach to implement improvement or quality care. It is important in such systematic approaches to pay particular attention to factors such as the credibility of the tool, individual motivation to use, compliance, leadership and cultural context, resources and expertise context, political and economic climate, as well as the structure of the implementation strategy of a tool (Sommerbakk *et al.* 2016). Practice development incorporates action learning promoting a continuing cycle of evaluation and improvement based on evidence and the practicalities of the clinical setting. To achieve a sustained, effective, evidence-based practice change requires a number of conditions working together.

Conditions identified as key to supporting effective, sustainable practice change include:

- *Recognising what change is needed and why:* Demonstrating that there is a discrepancy between the desired state and the current state of practice (Appelbaum and Wohl 2000).

- *Organisational and managerial commitment:* Giving time, resources and support. Organisations may respond to external change drivers such as health and social care policy or internal change drivers such as a critical incident review (Moran and Avergun 1997).

- *A change leader:* A member of staff who acts as a role model and works to generate interest and support among colleagues (Moran and Avergun 1997).

- *A change management team:* A group of individuals who interact interdependently and adaptively to achieve specified shared and valued objectives (Cameron and Green 2009). As internal change drivers, these individuals will have the most impact on practice at the client interface (Moran and Avergun 1997). Cameron and Green (2009) suggest that teamwork is paramount because of the level of work, energy and commitment needed to bring about change. Roberts, Nolet and Gatecliffe (2008) highlight the importance of working through a multidisciplinary team to effect change throughout an organisation.

- *Training:* To ensure that staff have the necessary knowledge and skills to implement the change (Pardo del Val and Martínez Fuentes 2003).

- *Communication:* Ensuring everyone is aware of the change and the systems by which it will be implemented while providing channels through which staff can express their thoughts and concerns about the development (Appelbaum and Wohl 2000).

- *Service user involvement:* To understand the person with dementia and their family's experience of any developments in the care they receive, with all practical steps taken to support the person with dementia to communicate their experience (Cheston, Bender and Byatt 2000).

The goal-setting theory (Locke and Latham 2002) emphasises that only small changes should be made at a time in a step-like approach to practice development. Each change needs to be:

- **S**pecific

- **M**easurable

- **A**chievable

- **R**ealistic

- **T**ime-bound.

The Claims, Concerns, Issues (CCI) exercise (McCormack, McCance and Maben 2013), derived from *Fourth Generation Evaluation* (see Guba and Lincoln 1989), is designed to gain the views and perspectives of all stakeholder groups involved with a project. This way, delivering change becomes a democratic process with which all parties remain engaged.

- *Claims:* Individuals are asked to identify favourable assertions about a project and its implementation.

- *Concerns:* Individuals are asked to identify unfavourable assertions about a project and its implementation.

- *Issues:* Questions that any reasonable person might ask about a project and its implementation. These usually arise out of the concerns.

This exercise can be used repeatedly with various stakeholder groups throughout the action learning process to highlight improvements achieved through a project and the difficulties remaining, and to develop an action plan to overcome the difficulties.

## Case study: Example from practice

A multidisciplinary group of hospice staff came together to respond to national policy and to address the concerns of staff around providing the appropriate care for patients with dementia. The group felt that it would be useful to ask the families of patients with dementia to support their relative in completing the 'This is me' leaflet (see Chapters 1 and 2). The group delivered workshops on 'the experience of dementia' that emphasised the importance of knowing as much as possible about the person with dementia in their care. The workshops evaluated well, and staff showed enthusiasm in promoting the use of the leaflet.

Initial evaluation of the initiative concluded that although most families of patients who were admitted to the hospice with dementia were offered a copy of the leaflet to complete, few gave sufficient information to impact on the care given. Of those that were completed in detail, the information was not accessed by all members of the multidisciplinary team, and did not appear to inform care plans.

Clinical staff of all disciplines were asked to complete a CCI exercise about using the 'This is me' leaflet. The views of patients and their relatives were also sought. Although everyone agreed that the principle was good, there were difficulties expressed around using the leaflet in practice. Some patients and families found it difficult to know what information would be useful; some found it difficult to think about such things when they were stressed by their situation; and for some, filling in a form was a challenge. The staff found it difficult to know how and when to approach the patients and families to ask them to complete the leaflet, and how to get all members of the multidisciplinary team to read it.

Through consultation with all the clinical teams, practical solutions were suggested to overcome the difficulties. To support the implementation of the leaflet into practice, the following was advocated:

- Staff should offer families and patients support to fill in the leaflet.

- The leaflet does not have to be completed in one go – some information may come as a result of conversations between the patient/family and the staff, and can be added at any time.

- A sticker put on the patient's notes could alert members of the multidisciplinary team that the leaflet is being used.

## TEAMWORKING

The interdisciplinary team (IDT), sometimes known as the interprofessional or multidisciplinary team, is recognised as a highly effective model of delivering the kind of integrated holistic care that individuals and their carers/families need at the end of life. The team comes in many forms. It may be based within specialist or community settings or may span both. It frequently involves a wide range of professionals, each bringing specialist as well as generalist skills and expertise – it is unrealistic to expect one service, profession or individual to have the skills to make the necessary assessment, institute the necessary interventions and provide ongoing monitoring.

The productivity of a team depends on relationships between individuals and the group dynamics of the team. Various factors influence the interactions and behaviours of teams including individual personalities, diversity of roles, differing levels of skill, experience, knowledge and commitment. The style of leadership is influential to the types of relationships that develop in teams. An open and inclusive style increases the likelihood of a mutually respectful climate within the group. A leader needs to notice and champion good practice and address poor practice to reduce the likelihood of a culture of complaining and scapegoating developing (Loveday 2012).

The National End of Life Care Programme (2013) has identified key issues for promoting effective interdisciplinary teamworking across the end of life care pathway. When coming into contact with an individual/carer at any point along the end of life care pathway, members of the IDT should consider the following:

- Does this person know who I am and what my role is in their care?

- What does this individual (and carer) know about their diagnosis and prognosis?

- What is this person's situation (including wishes/preferences, and relevant relationship dimensions, as well as their health status)?

- What really matters to this individual? How can I ensure this is communicated to others involved in their care?

- Who is the care coordinator/key worker, and who holds the information?

- Is there any documentation on this person?

- Who else is involved in caring for this individual? What other conversations have been had within the IDT? With the individual or carer? Might their needs or preferences have changed recently?

- Have my recommendations been followed through? Can I check?

- What other services are available within and outside my team, which this person could benefit from? Are my competences in this area up to date and at the correct level, and which referral protocols and policies apply in this situation?

- Who will I be handing over care to, and what information does that member of staff need to see in order to be able to provide the right care? Have I obtained informed consent to share this?

Issues that IDT managers should consider:

- How can we develop a culture of openness and shared personal and professional responsibility among all staff coming into contact with individuals nearing end of life?

- How can a culture of team decision-making be developed, avoiding a hierarchical approach where the expertise and insights of IDT or other non-'core' members of the team may not be fully utilised?

- Do our information-sharing systems meet the needs of the individual, carer and IDT, balancing convenience and the need for shared access against security and confidentiality requirements?

- Are adequate protocols in place for obtaining consent for sharing information, including between health and social care?

## SUPPORT FOR STAFF

Working with people with dementia can be intense, stressful and frightening (Loveday 2012). Others have noted how a lack of clinical leadership and supervision can contribute to poor-quality end of life care in nursing homes, arguing that adequate supervision of staff may enhance the quality of palliative care for people with dementia (Kayser-Jones *et al.* 2003). If staff are not adequately trained, they may inadvertently create stressful situations for people with dementia, resulting in challenging behaviour to manage. Equally staff may feel frustrated and exhausted, and experience strong personal feelings that can impact on their approach to care (Loveday 2012). Emerging evidence describes some of the heavy tolls experienced by health professionals who deal with the continual death of patients. Each patient and family has particular needs (physical, psychological, social and spiritual), and is deserving of expert end of life care, and it is this intensity of need that places professional carers at risk of compassion fatigue. There are clear physical and emotional health consequences for nurses who provide palliative care over extended periods of time (Melvin 2012).

The terms 'professional compassion fatigue' (PCF), 'burnout' and 'accumulated loss phenomenon' have all been used to refer to the cumulative physical and emotional effects of providing care over extended periods of time. These include anxiety, intrusive thoughts, apathy and depression (Slatten, Carson and Carson 2011). Loveday (2012) identifies that if dementia care staff do not receive sufficient support, the only way to manage their feelings is to construct a defensive barrier between themselves and those they care for, leading to an emotional disconnection that blocks empathy and inhibits relationships.

Jezuit (2003) determines that managers have a unique ability to assist nurses who are distressed as a result of repeated exposure to patient and family trauma and suffering. They must create a safe environment in which a nurse may express his/her distress and discuss methods to treat it. Similarly, Loveday (2012) emphasises that managers/leaders need to model how they want staff to be with the people they care for, and make it safe for staff to draw on their emotions and humanity to develop and sustain person-centred relationships by attending to the emotional needs of staff and work at developing trusting relationships with them. She suggests that leaders can provide emotional support for their staff by:

- making it clear they are there for staff to express their own feelings and willing to listen in a non-judgemental way

- showing interest and concern for personal problems experienced by their staff that are unrelated to work

- arranging formal one-to-one situations through clinical supervision and appraisal which are supportive, constructive and developmental, allowing staff to reflect on practice and to develop and share their ideas

- organising group support through team meetings, giving staff the opportunity for collaborative enquiry and creative thinking

- recognising staff who are experiencing grief as a result of personal or work-related experiences, and identifying those who would benefit from a referral for professional bereavement support.

## Case study: Staff self-awareness and support

Lisa has been working on the medical ward since first qualifying six years ago. The busy ward cares for patients with a variety of conditions, including patients admitted with dementia for treatment of other conditions such as chest infections. Lisa has always been a highly motivated and efficient nurse, noted for her ability to coordinate busy shifts and ensure that all patients are able to obtain the care that they need. Several staff have resigned recently and there have been problems recruiting. Lately, Lisa has been staying behind after her shift has ended to complete the care plans and administration.

She answers Wilfred's buzzer for the fourth time that afternoon – each time he has been unable to verbalise what he has needed and has seemed to settle with a smile and a kind word. She says to Wilfred, 'Please be patient – you're not the only patient on this ward and we will get to you as soon as we can.' Lisa returns to her paperwork and then goes home.

The following day she is called to speak to the ward sister. Wilfred's daughter arrived on the ward at visiting time and found her father in urine-soaked pyjamas, and asked to speak to the nurse in charge. The patient in the bed next door commented that he had been ringing his buzzer for hours and 'that nurse' just kept ignoring him because she was more concerned with her paperwork than anything else. Wilfred's daughter is livid and demands an explanation.

The ward sister calls Lisa and presents her with the story. Lisa tells her that she forgot he had been ringing because she had been so busy with coordinating the care plans. She feels that Wilfred is 'demanding and unreasonable' and 'does not seem to realise that there are other people than him'. She seems very angry but admits that she should have assessed Wilfred to see what the cause of his distress might be. She says, 'It's like the boy who cries wolf – when someone buzzes all the time, you get a bit immune to the sound.' She does agree to apologise to Wilfred and his daughter.

What can the ward sister do to support Lisa and to maintain high standards of care on her ward?

- She could help Lisa to reflect critically on the situation, helping her to recognise her own feelings towards Wilfred and to understand that his behaviour is an expression of unmet need.

- She could show her appreciation for the extra work that Lisa has put in, and reassure her that she is recognised as a valued team member with a good record of working efficiently.

- She could look at ways to help Lisa manage her workload – is there work she can delegate to others or can she be given dedicated time away from the ward to complete the administrative aspects of her role?

- She could identify whether Lisa has any training needs in relation to dementia care, and help her access the appropriate training.

- She could enquire about Lisa's emotional wellbeing – does she have any concerns at work or at home?

If the personhood of individual members of staff is not respected, they will find it difficult to practise person-centred care over an extended period of time, as it is an approach that relies on the building of authentic relationships. Nolan *et al.* (2004) developed the Senses Framework believing that all parties involved in caring – the cared for, family carers and formal carers – should experience relationships that promote a sense of security, continuity, belonging, purpose, achievement and significance. This Framework, considered earlier in relation to the cared for and family carers, is referred to here in relation to professional carers:

- Security:
  - To feel free from physical threat, rebuke or censure.
  - To have secure conditions of employment.
  - To have the emotional demands of work recognized, and to work within a supportive but challenging culture.

- Continuity:
  - Positive experience of work with older people from an early stage of their career.

- ○ Exposure to good role models and environments of care.

- ○ Expectations and standards of care communicated clearly and consistently.

- Belonging:

  - ○ To feel part of a team with a recognised and valued contribution.

  - ○ To belong to a peer group.

- Purpose:

  - ○ To have a sense of therapeutic direction, a clear set of goals to which to aspire.

- Achievement:

  - ○ To be able to provide good care.

  - ○ To feel satisfied with one's efforts.

  - ○ To contribute towards therapeutic goals as appropriate.

  - ○ To use skills and ability to the full.

- Significance:

  - ○ To feel one's practice is valued and one's work and effort 'matter'.

---

## Key points

- National policies, initiatives and resources are being implemented to support commissioners and managers determine the level of palliative and dementia care training required by individual staff, and to plan educational interventions in a variety of clinical settings to meet the needs of the vast workforce delivering palliative care to people with dementia.

- As well as effective training programmes, several other factors need to come together to enable an inclusive, sustained and targeted approach to implementing new knowledge into practice. These include leadership, interdisciplinary teamworking, listening to the views of people with dementia and their carers, and support from managers.

- Providing palliative care for people with dementia is demanding and emotionally challenging, and staff risk experiencing compassion fatigue if they do not receive the appropriate support from their leaders and managers. Leaders and managers need to be open and inclusive, act as role models and foster relationships of trust. Staff need to feel appreciated and valued as team members, have access to appropriate training, have supervision and support to engage with reflective practice, and freely express their ideas, concerns and feelings.

## ACKNOWLEDGEMENT

The authors wish to thank Dr Vanessa Taylor, Deputy Head of Nursing, Midwifery and Professional Programmes/Chair in Teaching and Learning at the University of York, for contributions to early drafts of Chapter 5.

# References

Agüero-Torres, H., Fratiglioni, L., Guo, Z., Viitanen, M. and Winblad, B. (1998) 'Prognostic factors in very old demented adults: A seven-year follow-up from a population-based survey in Stockholm.' *Journal of the American Geriatrics Society 46*, 444–452.

Ahmed, H.M.S. (2010) 'Hybrid e-learning acceptance model: Learner perceptions.' *Decision Sciences Journal of Innovative Education 8*, 2, 313–346.

Allan, K. and Killick, J. (2008) 'Communication and Relationships: An Inclusive Social World.' In M. Downs and B. Bowers (eds) *Excellence in Dementia Care: Research into Practice*. Maidenhead: Open University Press.

Alzheimer's Society (2012) *My Life Until the End: Dying Well with Dementia*. London: Alzheimer's Society.

Alzheimer's Society (no date) 'Caring for a person with dementia.' Available at www.alzheimers.org.uk/site/scripts/documents.php?categoryID=200343, accessed on 16 August 2016.

Andersen, E.A., Strumpel, C., Fensom, I. and Andrews, W. (2011) 'Implementing team based learning in large classes: Nurse educators' experiences.' *International Journal of Nursing Education Scholarship 8*, 2–19.

Appelbaum, S.H. and Wohl, L. (2000) 'Transformation or change: Some prescriptions for health care organizations.' *Managing Service Quality: An International Journal 10*, 5, 279–298.

APPG (All Party Parliamentary Group) on Dementia (2008) 'Always a last resort: *Inquiry into the prescription of antipsychotic drugs to people with dementia living in care homes*.' Available at www.publications.parliament.uk/pa/cm201012/cmselect/cmhealth/1430/1430we08.htm, accessed on 22 September 2016.

Ashida, S. (2000) 'The effect of reminiscence music therapy sessions on changes in depressive symptoms in elderly persons with dementia.' *Journal of Music Therapy 37*, 170–182.

Australian Commission on Safety and Quality in Health Care (2015) 'National consensus statement: Essential elements for safe and high-quality end-of-life care.' Available at www.safetyandquality.gov.au/wp-content/ uploads/2015/05/National-Consensus-Statement-Essential-Elements-forsafe-high-quality-end-of-life-care.pdf, accessed on 22 September 2016.

Badger, F., Plumridge, G., Hewison, A., Shaw, K.L., Thomas, K. and Clifford, C. (2012) 'An evaluation of the impact of the Gold Standards Framework on collaboration in end-of-life care in nursing homes: A qualitative and quantitative evaluation.' *International Journal of Nursing Studies 49*, 5, 586–595.

Baker, A., Leak, P. and Ritchie, L. (2012) 'Anticipatory care planning and integration: A primary care pilot study aimed at reducing unplanned hospitalisation.' *British Journal of General Practice 62*, 84–85.

Baldwin, C. (2008) 'Toward a Person-Centred Ethic in Dementia Care: Doing Right or Being Good?' In M. Downs and B. Bowers (eds) *Excellence in Dementia Care: Research into Practice*. Maidenhead: Open University Press.

Ballard, C. (2010) 'Which activities are most engaging for people with dementia living in care homes?' Available at www.alzheimers.org.uk/site/scripts/ download_info.php?fileID=1001, accessed on 22 September 2016.

Barnett, K., Mercer, S., Norbury, M., Watt, G., Wyke, S. and Guthrie, B. (2012) 'Epidemiology of multimorbidity and implications for health care, research, and medical education: A cross-sectional study.' *The Lancet 380*, 9836, 37–43.

Beauchamp, T. and Childress, J. (2001) *Principles of Biomedical Ethics*. Oxford: Oxford University Press.

Bennett, M. (2001) 'The LANSS Pain Scale: The Leeds assessment of neuropathic symptoms and signs.' *Pain 92*, 1, 147–157.

Birch, D. and Draper, J. (2008) 'A critical literature review exploring the challenges of delivering effective palliative care to older people with dementia.' *Journal of Clinical Nursing 17*, 1144–1163.

Black, J. (2011) 'Difficult conversations: Talking about dying well with dementia.' *British Journal of Neuroscience Nursing 7*, 617.

Booth, M., Springett, A., Nash, S. and Banks, C. (2014) 'Three approaches to delivering end-of-life education to care homes in a region of south east England.' *International Journal of Palliative Nursing 20*, 1, 18 February. Available at www.magonlinelibrary.com/doi/abs/10.12968/ ijpn.2014.20.1.27?url_ver=Z39.882003&rfr_id=ori:rid:crossref. org&rfr_dat=cr_pub%3dpubmed, accessed on 16 August 2016.

Bourgeois, M., Dijkstra, K., Burgio, L. and Allen-Burge, R. (2001) 'Memory aids as an augmentative and alternative communication strategy for nursing home residents with dementia.' *Augmentative and Alternative Communication 17*, 3, 196–210.

Bowlby, J. (1980) *Attachment and Loss: Loss, Sadness and Depression* (Vol. 3). New York: Basic Books.

Broad, M.L. (1997) 'Overview of transfer of training: From learning to performance.' *Performance Improvement Quarterly 10*, 2, 7–21.

Brodaty, H. and Donkin, M. (2009) 'Family caregivers of people with dementia.' *Dialogues in Clinical Neuroscience 11*, 2, 217–228.

Brodaty, H., Seeher, K. and Gibson, L. (2012) 'Dementia time to death: A systematic literature review on survival time and years of life lost in people with dementia.' *International Psychogeriatrics/IPA 24*, 1034–1045.

Brorson, H., Plymoth, H., Örmon, K. and Bolmsjö, I. (2014) 'Pain relief at the end of life: Nurses' experiences regarding end-of-life pain relief in patients with dementia.' *Pain Management Nursing 15*, 1, 315–323.

Brown, M.A., Sampson, E.L., Jones, L. and Barron, A.M. (2012) 'Prognostic indicators of 6-month mortality in elderly people with advanced dementia: A systematic review.' *Palliative Medicine.* 0269216312465649.

Buffum, M.D., Hutt, E., Chang, V.T., Craine, M.H. and Snow, A.L. (2007) 'Cognitive impairment and pain management: Review of issues and challenges.' *Journal of Rehabilitation Research and Development 44*, 2, 315.

BUPA (2010) [AQ]

Cameron, E. and Green, M. (2009) *Making Sense of Change Management: A Complete Guide to the Models, Tools and Techniques of Organizational Change.* London: Kogan Page Publishers.

Caron, C.D., Griffith, J. and Arcand, M. (2005) 'End-of-life decision making in dementia: The perspective of family caregivers.' *Dementia 4*, 1, 113–136.

Catt, S., Blanchard, M., Addington-Hall, J., Zis, M., Blizard, R. and King, M. (2005) 'Older adults' attitudes to death, palliative treatment and hospice care.' *Palliative Medicine 19*, 402–410.

Chang, E., Daly, J., Johnson, A., Harrison, K. *et al.* (2009) 'Challenges for professional care of advanced dementia.' *International Journal of Nursing Practice 15*, 1, 41–47.

Cheston, R., Bender, M. and Byatt, S. (2000) 'Involving people who have dementia in the evaluation of services: A review.' *Journal of Mental Health 9*, 5, 471–479.

Cohen, D. and Eisdorfer, C. (2002) *A Loss of Self: A Family Resource for the Care of Alzheimer's Disease and Related Disorders.* London: Norton & Company.

Collett, B., O'Mahoney, S., Schofield, P., Closs, S.J. and Potter, J. (2007) 'The assessment of pain in older people.' *Clinical Medicine 7*, 5, 496–500.

Collins, C., Liken, M., King, S. and Kokinakis, C. (1993) 'Loss and grief among family caregivers of relatives with dementia.' *Qualitative Health Research 3*, 2, 236–253.

Commission on Dignity in Care (2012) 'Delivering dignity: Securing dignity in care for older people in hospitals and care homes.' Available at www.nhsconfed.org/resources/2012/06/delivering-dignity-securing-dignity-in-care-for-older-people-in-hospitals-and-care, accessed on 9 August 2016.

Connell, C.M., Holmes, S.B., Voelkl, J.E. and Bakalar, H.R. (2002) 'Providing dementia outreach education to rural communities: Lessons learned from a train-the-trainer program.' *Journal of Applied Gerontology 21*, 3, 294–313.

Connolly, A., Sampson, E.L. and Purandare, N. (2012) 'End-of-life care for people with dementia from ethnic minority groups: A systematic review.' *Journal of the American Geriatrics Society 60*, 351–360.

Connor, H., Tyers, C., Modood, E. and Hillage, J. (2004) *Why the Difference? A Closer Look at Higher Education Minority Ethnic Students and Graduates.* Nottingham: Department for Education and Skills. Available at www.bristol.ac.uk/media-library/sites/ethnicity/migrated/documents/educationreport.pdf, accessed on 9 August 2016.

Cook, D.A., Levinson, A.J., Garside, S., Dupras, D.M., Erwin, P.J. and Montori, V.M. (2008) 'Internet-based learning in the health professions: A meta-analysis.' *Jama 300*, 10, 1181–1196.

Cook, M., Cook, E. and Driver, R. (2012) *Palliative and End of Life ABC Education Programme Impact Evaluation – Executive Summary*, July, 1–37. University of Bedfordshire.

Counsel and Care (1995) *Last Rites: A Study of How Death and Dying Are Handled in Residential Care and Nursing Homes.* London: Counsel and Care.

CQC (Care Quality Commission) (2013) 'Care update: March 2013.' Available at www.cqc.org.uk/sites/default/files/media/documents/cqc_care_update_issue_2.pdf, accessed on 23 July 2013.

CQC (2016) 'A different ending: Addressing inequalities in end of life care.' *Good Practice Case Studies.* Available at www.cqc.org.uk/content/different-ending-our-review-looking-end-life-care-published, accessed on 22 September 2016.

Cromwell, S.E. and Kolb, J.A. (2004) 'An examination of work-environment support factors affecting transfer of supervisory skills training to the workplace.' *Human Resource Development Quarterly 15*, 4, 449–471.

Curtiss, C.P. (2010) 'Challenges in pain assessment in cognitively intact and cognitively impaired older adults with cancer.' *Oncology Nursing Forum 37*, S7–16.

Deno, M., Tashiro, M., Miyashita, M., Asakage, T. *et al.* (2012) 'The mediating effects of social support and self-efficacy on the relationship between social distress and emotional distress in head and neck cancer outpatients with facial disfigurement.' *Psycho-Oncology 21*, 144–152.

DeWaters, T., Popovitch, J. and Faut-Callahan, M. (2003) 'An evaluation of clinical tools to measure pain in older people with cognitive impairment.' *British Journal of Community Nursing 8*, 5, 226–234.

Dewing, J. (2009) 'Caring for people with dementia: Noise and light.' *Nursing Older People 21*, 34–38.

DH (Department of Health) (2008a) *End of Life Care Strategy: Promoting High Quality Care for All Adults at the End of Life.* London: DH.

DH (2008b) *Carers at the Heart of 21st-Century Families and Communities: 'A Caring System on Your Side. A Life of Your Own.'* London: HM Government.

DH (2009a) *The Mental Capacity Act Deprivation of Liberty Safeguards.* London: DH.

DH (2009b) *Living Well with Dementia: A National Dementia Strategy.* February. London: DH.

DH (2011) *Independent Palliative Care Funding Review.* 1 July. London: DH. Available at www.gov.uk/government/publications/independent-palliative-care-funding-review, accessed on 16 August 2016.

DH (2015) *Delivering High Quality, Effective, Compassionate Care: Developing the Right People with the Right Skills and the Right Value. A Mandate from the Government to Health Education England: April 2015 to March 2016.* Leeds: DH. Available at www.gov.uk/government/uploads/system/uploads/attachment_data/file/411200/HEE_Mandate.pdf, accessed on 22 September 2016.

Downs, M., Small, N. and Froggatt, N. (2006) 'Explanatory models of dementia: Links to end-of-life care.' *International Journal of Palliative Nursing 12,* 5, 209–213.

Dying Matters (2012) *Dying to Know* [film]. London: Dying Matters.

Ellis-Smith, C., Evans, C.J., Bone, A.E., Henson, L.A. *et al.* (2016) 'Measures to assess commonly experienced symptoms for people with dementia in long-term care settings: A systematic review.' *BMC Medicine 14,* 38. Available at www.ncbi.nlm.nih.gov/pmc/articles/PMC4769567, accessed on 16 August 2016.

Evans, C. and Goodman, C. (2009) 'Changing practice in dementia care for people in care homes towards the end of life.' *Dementia 8,* 424–431.

Fabbro, E.D., Dalal, S. and Bruera, E. (2006) 'Symptom control in palliative care – Part II: Cachexia/anorexia and fatigue.' *Journal of Palliative Medicine 9,* 2, 409–421.

Farrington, C.J. (2014) 'Blended e-learning and end of life care in nursing homes: A small-scale mixed-methods case study.' *BMC Palliative Care 13,* 1, 31. Available at www.biomedcentral.com/1472-684X/13/31, accessed on 22 September 2016.

Fick, D.M., Agostini, J.V. and Inouye, S.K. (2002) 'Delirium superimposed on dementia: A systematic review.' *Journal of the American Geriatrics Society 50,* 10, 1723–1732.

Finucane, T.E., Christmas, C. and Travis, K. (1999) 'Tube feeding in patients with advanced dementia: A review of the evidence.' *Journal of American Geriatric Society 282,* 14, 1365–1370.

Folkman, S., Lazarus, R.S., Gruen, R.J. and DeLongis, A. (1986) 'Appraisal, coping, health status, and psychological symptoms.' *Journal of Personality and Social Psychology 50,* 3, 571.

Fong, T.G., Davis, D., Growdon, M.E., Albuquerque, A. and Inouye, S.K. (2015) 'The interface between delirium and dementia in elderly adults.' *Lancet Neurology 14*, 8, 823–832. Available at www.ncbi.nlm.nih.gov/pubmed/26139023, accessed on 16 August 2016.

Forbes, S., Bern-Klug, M. and Gessert, C. (2000) 'End-of-life decision making for nursing home residents with dementia.' *Journal of Nursing Scholarship 32*, 3, 251–258.

Gallagher, A., Li, S., Wainwright, P., Jones, I. and Lee, D. (2008) 'Dignity in the care of older people – A review of the theoretical and empirical literature.' *BMC Nursing 7*, 11.

Gamondi, C., Larkin, P. and Payne, S. (2013a) 'Core competencies in palliative care: An EAPC white paper on palliative care education. Part 1. *European Journal of Palliative Care 20*, 2, 86–91.

Gamondi, C., Larkin, P. and Payne, S. (2013b) 'Core competencies in palliative care: An EAPC white paper on palliative care education. Part 2. *European Journal of Palliative Care 20*, 3, 140–145.

Gawande, A. (2014) *Being Mortal: Medicine and What Matters in the End.* New York: Metropolitan Books, Henry Holt and Company.

Gethin, G. (2012) 'Understanding the inflammatory process in wound healing.' *British Journal of Community Nursing 17*, S17–22.

Ghiotti, C. (2009) 'The Dementia End of Life Care Project (DeLCaP): Supporting families caring for people with late stage dementia at home.' *Dementia 8*, 3, 349–361.

Gibbons, L. (2012) 'A carer's confession.' Available at www.alzheimers readingroom.com, accessed on 16 August 2016.

Gibbs, G. (1988) *Learning by Doing: A Guide to Learning and Teaching Methods.* Birmingham: SCED.

Gijsberts, M.-J., van der Steen, J.T., Muller, M.T., Hertogh, C.M. and Deliens, L. (2013) 'Spiritual end-of-life care in Dutch nursing homes: An ethnographic study.' *Journal of the American Medical Directors Association 14*, 679–684.

Gillick, M.R. (2000) 'Rethinking the role of tube feeding in patients with advanced dementia.' *New England Journal of Medicine – Unbound Volume 342*, 3, 206–210.

GMC (General Medical Council) (2010) *Treatment and Care Towards the End of Life: Good Practice in Decision Making.* London: GMC. Available at www.gmc-uk. org/End_of_life.pdf_32486688.pdf, accessed on 16 August 2016.

Goodman, C., Dening, T., Gordon, A.L., Davies, S.L. *et al.* (2016) 'Effective health care for older people living and dying in care homes: A realist review.' *BMC Health Services Research 16*, 1, 269.

Goodman, C., Drennan, V., Scheibl, F., Shah, D. *et al.* (2011) 'Models of inter professional working for older people living at home: A survey and review of the local strategies of English health and social care statutory organisations.' *BMC Health Services Research 11*, 1, 1.

Gott, M., Seymour, J., Ingleton, C., Gardiner, C. *et al.* (2012) '"That's part of everybody's job": The perspectives of health care staff in England and New Zealand on the meaning and remit of palliative care.' *Palliative Medicine 26,* 3, 232–241.

Grande, G. and Keady, J. (2011) 'Needs, Access, and Support for Older Carers.' In M. Gott and C. Ingleton (eds) *Living with Ageing and Dying: Palliative and End of Life Care in Older People.* Oxford: Oxford University Press.

Greenhalgh, T. (2001) 'Computer assisted learning in undergraduate medical education.' *BMJ (Clinical Research ed.) 322,* 7277, 40–44.

Guba, E.G. and Lincoln, Y.S. (1989) *Fourth Generation Evaluation.* Newbury Park, CA, London and Delhi: Sage Publications.

Hadjistavropoulos, T., Fitzgerald, T.D. and Marchildon, G.P. (2010) 'Practice guidelines for assessing pain in older persons with dementia residing in long-term care facilities.' *Physiotherapy Canada 62,* 2, 104– 113.

Hadjistavropoulos, T., Voyer, P., Sharpe, D., Verreault, R. and Aubin, M. (2008) 'Assessing pain in dementia patients with comorbid delirium and/or depression.' *Pain Management Nursing 9,* 2, 48–54.

Hall, S., Kolliakou, A., Petkova, H., Froggatt, K. and Higginson, I.J. (2011) 'Interventions for improving palliative care for older people living in nursing care homes.' *Cochrane Database of Systematic Reviews.*

Hanratty, B., Lowson, E., Grande, G., Payne, S. *et al.* (2014) 'Transitions at the end of life for older adults – Patient, carer and professional perspectives: A mixed-methods study.' *Health Services and Delivery Research 2,* 17. Available at www.ncbi.nlm.nih.gov/books/NBK263541, accessed on 9 August 2016.

Hardy, I.J. (2012) 'Researching professional educational practice: The case for "dirty theory".' *Educational Theory 62,* 517–533.

Harper, L. (2013) 'The spiritual implications of dementia.' *Huffington Post.* 14 July. Available at www.huffingtonpost.com/lynn-casteel-harper/the-spiritual-implication_b_644586.html, accessed on 16 August 2016.

Harrison Dening, K., Greenish, W., Jones, L., Mandal, U. and Sampson, E.L. (2012) 'Barriers to providing end-of-life care for people with dementia: A whole-system qualitative study.' *BMJ Supportive and Palliative Care 2,* 103–107.

Harrison Dening, K., Jones, L. and Sampson, E.L. (2013) 'Preferences for end-of-life care: A nominal group study of people with dementia and their family carers.' *Palliative Medicine 27,* 5, 409–417. Available at www.ncbi.nlm.nih.gov/pubmed/23128905, accessed on 16 August 2016.

Harrison Dening, K., King, M., Jones, L., Vickestaff, V. and Sampson, E.L. (2016) 'Advance care planning in dementia: Do family carers know the treatment preferences of people with early dementia?' *PLoS One 11,* 7. Available at www.ncbi.nlm.nih.gov/pubmed/27410259, accessed on 16 August 2016.

Hendrix, C.C., Sakauye, K.M., Karabatsos, G. and Daigle, D. (2003) 'The use of the minimum data set to identify depression in the elderly.' *Journal of the American Medical Directors Association 4*, 6, 308–312.

Hennings, J., Froggatt, K. and Keady, J. (2010) 'Approaching the end of life and dying with dementia in care homes: The accounts of family carers.' *Reviews in Clinical Gerontology 20*, 114–127.

Hennings, J., Froggatt, K. and Payne, S. (2013) 'Spouse caregivers of people with advanced dementia in nursing homes: A longitudinal narrative study.' *Palliative Medicine.* 0269216313479685.

Herr, K., Spratt, K.F., Garand, L. and Li, L. (2007) 'Evaluation of the Iowa pain thermometer and other selected pain intensity scales in younger and older adult cohorts using controlled clinical pain: A preliminary study.' *Pain Medicine 8*, 7, 585–600.

Hockley, J. (2014) 'Learning, support and communication for staff in care homes: Outcomes of reflective debriefing groups in two care homes to enhance end-of-life care.' *International Journal of Older People Nursing 9*, 2, 118–130.

Hockley, J., Watson, J., Oxenham, D. and Murray, S.A. (2010) 'The integrated implementation of two end-of-life care tools in nursing care homes in the UK: An in-depth evaluation.' *Palliative Medicine 24*, 828–838.

Hodges, E. (2015) 'Developing hospice services for people living with dementia.' Available at www.ehospice.com/uk/ArticleView/tabid/10697/ArticleId /14503/language/en-GB/View.aspx, accessed on 16 August 2016.

Hofman, A., Rocca, W., Brayne, C., Breteler, M. *et al.* (1991) 'The prevalence of dementia in Europe: A collaborative study of 1980–1990 findings.' Eurodem Prevalence Research Group. *International Journal of Epidemiology 20*, 736–748.

Hope, T. (2009) 'Ethical dilemmas in the care of people with dementia.' *British Journal of Community Nursing 14*, 12, 548–550.

Hospice UK (2015) 'Hospice enabled dementia care: The first steps. A guide to help hospices establish care for people with dementia, their families and carers.' Available at www.hospiceuk.org/what-we-offer/clinical-and-care-support/hospice-enabled-dementia-care, accessed on 22 September 2016.

Hospice UK (no date) 'Hospice enabled dementia care: What we offer.' Available at www.hospiceuk.org/what-we-offer/clinical-and-care-support/hospice-enabled-dementia-care, accessed on 16 August 2016.

Hughes, J., Jolley, D., Jordan, A. and Sampson, E. (2007) 'Palliative care in dementia: Issues and evidence.' *Advances in Psychiatric Treatment 13*, 251–260.

Hui, D., Mori, M., Parsons, H.A., Kim, S.H. *et al.* (2012) 'The lack of standard definitions in the supportive and palliative oncology literature.' *Journal of Pain and Symptom Management 43*, 582–592.

Hurley, A.C., Volicer, B.J. and Volicer, L. (1996) 'Effect of fever-management strategy on the progression of dementia of the Alzheimer type.' *Alzheimer Disease & Associated Disorders 10*, 1, 5–10.

Husebo, B.S., Achterberg, W. and Po, E. (2016) 'Identifying and managing pain in people with Alzheimer's disease and other types of dementia: A systematic review.' *CNS Drugs 30*, 418–497. Available at www.ncbi.nlm. nih.gov/pmc/articles/PMC4920848, accessed on 9 August 2016.

Independent Commission on Dignity in Care (2012) 'Delivering dignity: Securing dignity in care for older people in hospitals and care homes.' Available at www.nhsconfed.org/~/media/Confederation/Files/Publications/ Documents/Delivering_Dignity_final_report150612.pdf, accessed on 22 September 2016.

Ingvorsen, A. (2013) 'Guilty as charged.' Available at http://ingvorsen. wordpress.com/2013/02/25/dementia-concerns-jpg, accessed on 16 August 2016.

Jezuit, D. (2003) 'Personalization as it relates to nurse suffering: How managers can recognize the phenomenon and assist suffering nurses.' *JONA's Healthcare Law, Ethics and Regulation 5*, 2, 25–28.

Johnston, B. and Narayanasamy, M. (2016) 'Exploring psychosocial interventions for people with dementia that enhance personhood and relate to legacy: An integrative review.' *BMC Geriatrics 16*, 77. Available at www.ncbi.nlm. nih.gov/pmc/articles/PMC4820853, accessed on 16 August 2016.

Jordan, A., Regnard, C., O'Brien, J.T. and Hughes, J.C. (2012) 'Pain and distress in advanced dementia: Choosing the right tools for the job.' *Palliative Medicine 26*, 7, 873–878.

Kant, I. (1967) *Critique of Practical Reason, and Other Works on the Theory of Ethics.* Harlow: Longman.

Kayser-Jones, J., Schell, E., Lyons, W., Kris, A.E., Chan, J. and Beard, R.L. (2003) 'Factors that influence end-of-life care in nursing homes: The physical environment, inadequate staffing, and lack of supervision.' *The Gerontologist 43* (suppl. 2), 76–84.

Keele, K.D. (1948) 'The pain chart.' *Lancet 2*, 6514, 6–8.

Kennedy, C., Brooks-Young, P., Gray, C.B., Larkin, P. *et al.* (2014) 'Diagnosing dying: An integrative literature review.' *BMJ Supportive and Palliative Care 4*, 3, 263–270.

Kitwood, T. (1990) 'The dialectics of dementia: With particular reference to Alzheimer's disease.' *Ageing and Society 10*, 2, 177–196.

Kitwood, T. (1997) *Dementia Reconsidered: The Person Comes First.* Buckingham: Open University Press.

Kolb, D.A. (1984) *Experiential Learning: Experience as the Source of Learning and Development* (Vol. 1). Englewood Cliffs: Prentice-Hall.

Kovach, C.R., Weissman, D.E., Griffie, J., Matson, S. and Muchka, S. (1999) 'Assessment and treatment of discomfort for people with late-stage dementia.' *Journal of Pain and Symptom Management 18*, 6, 412–419.

Kremer, E., Atkinson, J.H. and Ignelzi, R.J. (1981) 'Measurement of pain: Patient preference does not confound pain measurement.' *Pain 10*, 2, 241–248.

Kübler-Ross, E. (1969) *On Death and Dying*. New York: Macmillan.

Kupeli, N., Leavey, G., Harrington, J., Lord, K. *et al.* (2016a) 'What are the barriers to care integration for those at the advanced stages of dementia living in care homes in the UK? Health care professional perspective.' *Dementia*. Available at www.ncbi.nlm.nih.gov/pubmed/26935834, accessed on 22 September 2016.

Kupeli, N., Leavey, G., Moore, K., Harrington, J. *et al.* (2016b) 'Context, mechanisms and outcomes in end of life care for people with advanced dementia.' *BMC Palliative Care 15*, 1, 1.

Lavoie, M., Blondeau, D. and de Koninck, T. (2008) 'The dying person: An existential being until the end of life.' *Nursing Philosophy 9*, 89–97.

Lawlor, P.G., Fainsinger, R.L. and Bruera, E.D. (2000) 'Delirium at the end of life: Critical issues in clinical practice and research.' *JAMA 284*, 19, 2427–2429.

Lawrence, R.M. (2003) 'Aspects of Spirituality in Dementia Care: When Clinicians Tune into Silence.' *Dementia 2*, 3, 393–402.

Lawrence, V., Samsi, K., Murray, J., Harari, D. and Banerjee, S. (2011) 'Dying well with dementia: qualitative examination of end-of-life care.' *British Journal of Psychiatry 199*, 5, 417–422.

Leadership Alliance for the Care of Dying People (2014) 'One chance to get it right: Improving people's experience of care in the last few days and hours of life.' Available at www.gov.uk/government/uploads/system/uploads/attachment_data/file/323188/One_chance_to_get_it_right.pdf, accessed on 16 August 2016.

Lichtner, V., Dowding, D., Allcock, N., Keady, J. *et al.* (2016) 'The assessment and management of pain in patients with dementia in hospital settings: A multi-case exploratory study from a decision making perspective.' *BMC Health Services Research 16*, 1, 427.

Liu, L., Guarino, A. and Lopez, R. (2011) 'Family satisfaction with care provided by nurse practitioners to nursing home residents with dementia at the end of life.' *Clinical Nursing Research 21*, 350–367.

Locke, E.A. and Latham, G.P. (2002) 'Building a practically useful theory of goal setting and task motivation: A 35-year odyssey.' *American Psychologist 57*, 9, 705.

Lorem, G. (2005) 'Withdrawal and exclusion: A study of the spoken word as means of understanding schizophrenic patients.' Doctoral thesis, University of Tromsø, Norway.

Love, A.W. (2007) 'Progress in understanding grief, complicated grief, and caring for the bereaved.' *Contemporary Nurse: A Journal for the Australian Nursing Profession 27*, 73–83.

Loveday, B. (2012) *Leadership for Person-Centred Dementia Care*. London: Jessica Kingsley Publishers.

Lyketsos, C.G., Lopez, O., Jones, B., Fitzpatrick, A.L., Breitner, J. and DeKosky, S. (2002) 'Prevalence of neuropsychiatric symptoms in dementia and mild cognitive impairment: Results from the cardiovascular health study.' *JAMA 288*, 12, 1475–1483.

Lynn, J. and Adamson, D.M. (2003) *Living Well at the End of Life: Adapting Health Care to Serious Chronic Illness in Old Age.* Santa Monica, CA: Rand Corp.

Maben, J., Latter, S. and Macleod Clark, J. (2006) 'The theory–practice gap: Impact of professional-bureaucratic work conflict on newly-qualified nurses.' *Journal of Advanced Nursing 55*, 465–477.

Magee, C. and Koffman, J. (2014) 'Supporting general practitioners to provide out-of-hours palliative care.' *BMJ Supportive and Palliative Care 4*, 1, 107.

Manley, K. (2005) *Changing Patients' Worlds through Nursing Practice Expertise: Exploring Nursing Practice Expertise through Emancipatory Action Research and Fourth Generation Evaluation.* London: RCN.

Maslow, A.H. (1943) *Motivation and Personality.* New York: Harper.

McCabe, M., You, E. and Tatangelo, G. (2016) 'Hearing their voice: A systematic review of dementia family caregivers' needs.' *Gerontologist.* 21 April. Available at www.ncbi.nlm.nih.gov/pubmed/27102056, accessed on 16 August 2016.

McCaffery, M. (1968) *N-110B Clinical Nursing: Nursing Practice Theories Related to Cognition, Bodily Pain, and Man–Environment Interactions.* Regents of the University of California.

McCarthy, M., Addington-Hall, J. and Altmann, D. (1997) 'The experience of dying with dementia: A retrospective study.' *International Journal of Geriatric Psychiatry 12*, 3, 404–409.

McCormack, B. (2003) 'A conceptual framework for person-centred practice with older people.' *International Journal of Nursing Practice 9*, 202–209.

McCormack, B., McCance, T. and Maben, J. (2013) 'Outcome Evaluation in the Development of Person-Centred Practice.' In B. McCormack, K. Manley and A. Titchen (eds) *Practice Development in Nursing and Healthcare.* London: John Wiley & Sons.

Meier, D.E., Ahronheim, J.C., Morris, J., Baskin-Lyons, S. and Morrison, R.S. (2001) 'High short-term mortality in hospitalized patients with advanced dementia: lack of benefit of tube feeding.' *Archives of Internal Medicine 161*, 4, 594–599.

Melvin, C.S. (2012) 'Professional compassion fatigue: What is the true cost of nurses caring for the dying?' *International Journal of Palliative Nursing 18*, 12, 606–611.

Melzack, R. (1987) 'The short-form McGill Pain Questionnaire.' *Pain 30*, 2, 191–197.

Melzack, R. and Wall, P.D. (1967) 'Pain mechanisms: A new theory.' *Survey of Anesthesiology 11*, 2, 89–90.

Mental Capacity Act (2005) *Code of Practice.* Department for Constitutional Affairs. London: TSO.

Michaelson, L., Knight, A. and Fink, L. (2002) *Team-Based Learning: A Transformative Use of Small Groups.* New York: Praeger.

Mitchell, S.L., Kiely, D.K. and Hamel, M.B. (2004) 'Dying with advanced dementia in the nursing home.' *Archives of Internal Medicine 164,* 3, 321–326.

Mitchell, S.L., Teno, J.M., Kiely, D.K., Shaffer, M.L. *et al.* (2009) 'The clinical course of advanced dementia.' *New England Journal of Medicine 361,* 1529–1538.

Moran, J. and Avergun, A. (1997) 'Creating lasting change.' *The TQM Magazine 9,* 2, 146–151.

Morrison, S.A.L. and Siu, A. (2000) 'Survival in end-stage dementia following acute illness.' *JAMA 284,* 47–52.

Moss, A.H., Lunney, J.R., Culp, S., Auber, M. *et al.* (2010) 'Prognostic significance of the "surprise" question in cancer patients.' *Journal of Palliative Medicine 13,* 837–840.

Murphy, J., Gray, C.M. and Cox, S. (2007) *Using 'Talking Mats' to Help People with Dementia to Communicate.* York: Joseph Rowntree Foundation.

Murray, S. and McLoughlin, P. (2012) 'Illness Trajectories and Palliative Care: Implications for Holistic Service Provision for All in the Last Day of Life.' In L. Sallnow, S. Kumar and A. Kellehear (eds) *International Perspectives on Public Health and Palliative Care.* London: Routledge.

Murtagh, F. (2013) 'Foreword.' In S. Payne, N. Preston, M. Turner and L. Rolls, *Research in Palliative Care: Can Hospices Afford Not to Be Involved?* A report for the Commission into the Future of Hospice Care.

National Palliative and End of Life Care Partnership (2015) 'Ambitions for palliative and end of life care: A national framework for local action 2015–2020.' Available at http://endoflifecareambitions.org.uk/wp-content/uploads/2015/09/Ambitions-for-Palliative-and-End-of-Life-Care.pdf, accessed on 16 August 2016.

NCPC (The National Council for Palliative Care) (2009) *The Power of Partnership: Palliative Care in Dementia.* London: NCPC. Available at https://palliativecarenwpctl.wordpress.com/2010/01/27/the-power-of-partnership-palliative-care-in-dementia, accessed on 16 August 2016.

NCPC (2011) *Difficult Conversations for Dementia.* London: NCPC.

NCPC (2012) *How Would I Know? What Can I Do?* London: NCPC. Available at www.ncpc.org.uk/news/how-would-i-know-what-can-i-do, accessed on 16 August 2016.

NEoLCP (National End of Life Care Programme) (2009) *Common Core Competences and Principles for Health and Social Care Workers Working with Adults at the End of Life.* London: National End of Life Care Intelligence Network (NEoLCIN).

NEoLCP (2010) *Deaths from Alzheimer's Disease, Dementia and Senility in England.* London: National End of Life Care Intelligence Network (NEoLCIN).

NEoLCP (2013) 'Optimising the role and value of the interdisciplinary team: Providing person-centred end of life care.' Available at http://socialwelfare.bl.uk/subject-areas/services-activity/health-services/nhsnationalendoflifecareprogramme/146158EoLC_IDT_Guide_Final[1].pdf, accessed on 22 September 2016.

Neuberger, J., Aaronovitch, D., Hameed, K., Bonser, T. *et al.* (2013) *More Care, Less Pathway: A Review of the Liverpool Care Pathway.* London: Independent Review of the Liverpool Care Pathway. Available at www.gov.uk/government/uploads/system/uploads/attachment_data/file/212450/Liverpool_Care_Pathway.pdf, accessed on 22 September 2016.

NHS England (2011) *Preferred Priorities for Care.* London: NHS England. Available at www.nhsiq.nhs.uk/resource-search/publications/eolc-ppc.aspx, accessed on 16 August 2016.

NHS Finance and Operations/NHS Group/NHS Clinical Services (2016) *Our Commitment to You for End of Life Care: The Government Response to the Review of Choice in End of Life Care.* July. London: Department of Health. Available at www.gov.uk/government/uploads/system/uploads/attachment_data/file/536326/choice-response.pdf, accessed on 16 July 2016.

NICE (National Institute for Health and Care Excellence) (2010) *Delirium. Pre-Delirium: Prevention, Diagnosis and Management.* Clinical Guideline 103. London: NICE. Available at www.nice.org.uk/guidance/cg103, accessed on 22 September 2016.

NICE (2011) *End of Life Care for Adults.* Quality Standard 13. London: NICE. Available at www.nice.org.uk/guidance/qs13, accessed on 16 August 2016.

NICE (2015) *Care of Dying Adults in the Last Days of Life.* NICE Guideline 31. December. London: NICE. Available at www.nice.org.uk/guidance/ng31, accessed on 17 August 2016.

NICE (2016) *Dementia: Supporting People with Dementia and Their Carers in Health and Social Care.* Clinical Guideline 42 (updated May 2016). London: NICE. Available at www.nice.org.uk/guidance/cg42, accessed on 22 September 2016.

Nolan, M. and Ryan, T. (2011) 'Family Carers, Palliative Care and the End-of-Life.' In M. Gott and C. Ingleton (eds) *Living with Ageing and Dying: Palliative and End of Life Care for Older People.* Oxford: Oxford University Press.

Nolan, M., Davies, S., Brown, J., Keady, J. and Nolan, J. (2004) 'Beyond "person-centred" care: A new vision for gerontological nursing.' *Journal of Clinical Nursing 13* (suppl. 1), 45–53.

Nordenfelt, L. (2004) 'The varieties of dignity.' *Health Care Analysis 12,* 69–81.

O'Callaghan, A., Laking, G., Frey, R., Robinson, J. and Gott, M. (2014) 'Can we predict which hospitalised patients are in their last year of life? A prospective cross-sectional study of the Gold Standards Framework Prognostic Indicator Guidance as a screening tool in the acute hospital setting.' *Palliative Medicine.* 0269216314536089.

Ødbehr, L.S., Hauge, S., Danbolt, L.J. and Kvigne, K. (2015) 'Residents' and caregivers' views on spiritual care and their understanding of spiritual needs in persons with dementia: A meta-synthesis.' *Dementia.* 30 December. Available at www.ncbi.nlm.nih.gov/pubmed/26721285, accessed on 16 August 2016.

Olson, E.I.M. (2003) 'Dementia and Neurodegenerative Diseases.' In R. Morrison, D. Meier and C. Capello (eds) *Geriatric Palliative Care.* New York: Oxford University Press.

ONS (2013) 'National Survey of Bereaved People (VOICES): 2013. Quality of care for people with dementia contributing to death.' Available at www.ons.gov.uk/peoplepopulationandcommunity/healthandsocialcare/healthcaresystem/bulletins/nationalsurveyofbereavedpeoplevoices/2014-07-10#quality-of-care-for-people-with-dementia-contributing-to-death, accessed on 12 October 2016.

ONS (2015) 'Life expectancy at birth and at age 65 for the UK and constituent countries.' *Dataset.* 16 April. Available at www.ons.gov.uk/peoplepopulationandcommunity/birthsdeathsandmarriages/lifeexpectancies/datasets/lifeexpectancyatbirthandatage65bylocalareasintheunitedkingdomtable4ukandconstituentcountries, accessed on 12 August 2016.

ONS (2016) 'National Survey of Bereaved People (VOICES): England, 2015. Quality of care delivered in the last 3 months of life for adults who died in England.' Available at www.ons.gov.uk/peoplepopulationandcommunity/healthandsocialcare/healthcaresystem/bulletins/nationalsurveyofbereavedpeoplevoices/england2015, accessed on 22 September 2016.

Owen, J.E., Goode, K.T. and Haley, W.E. (2001) 'End of life care and reactions to death in African-American and white family caregivers of relatives with Alzheimer's disease.' *OMEGA – Journal of Death and Dying 43,* 4, 349–361.

Oyebode, J. (2008) 'Grief and Bereavement.' In M. Downs and B. Bowers (eds) *Excellence in Dementia Care: Research into Practice.* Maidenhead: Open University Press.

Pardo del Val, M. and Martínez Fuentes, C. (2003) 'Resistance to change: A literature review and empirical study.' *Management Decision 41,* 2, 148–155.

Parkes, C.M. (1976) 'Determinants of outcome following bereavement.' *OMEGA – Journal of Death and Dying 6,* 4, 303–323.

Payne, S., Horn, S. and Relf, M. (1999) *Health Psychology: Loss and Bereavement.* Buckingham: Open University Press.

Peacock, S., Forbes, D., Markle-Reid, M., Hawranik, P. et al. (2009) 'The positive aspects of the caregiving journey with dementia: Using a strengths-based perspective to reveal opportunities.' *Journal of Applied Gerontology 29,* 5, 640–659.

Peacock, S., Bayly, M., Gibson, K., Holtslander, L., Thompson, G. and O'Connell, M. (2016) 'The bereavement experience of spousal caregivers to persons with dementia: Reclaiming self.' *Dementia.* 17 February. Available at www. ncbi.nlm.nih.gov/pubmed/26892303, accessed on 16 August 2016.

Pearlin, L.I., Mullan, J.T., Semple, S.J. and Skaff, M.M. (1990) 'Caregiving and the stress process: An overview of concepts and their measures.' *The Gerontologist 30,* 5, 583–594.

Poblador-Plou, B., Calderón-Larrañaga, A., Marta-Moreno, J., Hancco-Saavedra, J. *et al.* (2014) 'Comorbidity of dementia: A cross-sectional study of primary care older patients.' *BMC Psychiatry 14,* 84.

Prince, M., Knapp, M., Guerchet, M., McCrone, P. *et al.* (2014) *Dementia UK: Update* (2nd edn). Alzheimer's Society. Available at www.alzheimers.org. uk/site/scripts/documents_info.php?documentID=412, accessed on 22 September 2016.

Puchalski, C.M., Lunsford, B., Harris, M.H. and Miller, R.T. (2006) 'Interdisciplinary spiritual care for seriously ill and dying patients: A collaborative model.' *Cancer Journal 12,* 398–416.

Pyper, T., Sawyer, J., Pyper, C. and Mayhew, L. (2013) 'Summary of PHAST evaluation of three end of life care training pilots in the east of England.' Available at www.phast.org.uk, accessed on 22 September 2016.

Rawlinson, F. and Luyirika, E. (2014) 'Collaboration across continents to produce e-learning for palliative care education in Sub Saharan Africa.' *eCancer Medical Science 8,* ed36.

RCN (Royal College of Nursing) (2011) 'Dignity in dementia: Transforming general hospital care. Summary of findings from survey of professionals.' Available at www2.rcn.org.uk/__data/assets/pdf_file/0019/405109/RCN_Dementia_project_professional_survey_findings_.pdf, accessed on 22 September 2016.

Regnard, C. and Huntley, M.E. (2006) 'Managing the Physical Symptoms of Dying.' In J.C. Hughes (ed.) *Palliative Care in Severe Dementia.* London: Quay Books.

Regnard, C., Reynolds, J., Watson, B., Matthews, D., Gibson, L. and Clarke, C. (2007) 'Understanding distress in people with severe communication difficulties: Developing and assessing the Disability Distress Assessment Tool (DisDAT).' *Journal of Intellectual Disability Research 51,* 4, 277–292.

Resuscitation Council (2016) 'Do not attempt CPR.' Available at www.resus. org.uk/dnacpr/decisions-relating-to-cpr, accessed on 16 August 2016.

Rewston, C. and Moniz-Cook, E. (2008) 'Understanding and Alleviating Emotional Distress.' In M. Downs and B. Bowers (eds) *Excellence in Dementia Care: Research into Practice.* Maidenhead: Open University Press.

Roberts, T., Nolet, K. and Gatecliffe, L. (2008) 'Leadership in Dementia Care.' In M. Downs and B. Bowers (eds) *Excellence in Dementia Care: Research into Practice.* Maidenhead: Open University Press.

Robertson, P. (2001) 'Music and Health.' In A. Dilani (ed.) *Design and Health – The Therapeutic Benefits of Design.* Stockholm: Elanders Svenskt Tryck AB.

Robinson, L., Dickinson, C., Rousseau, N., Beyer, F. *et al.* (2012) 'A systematic review of the effectiveness of advance care planning interventions for people with cognitive impairment and dementia.' *Age and Ageing 41,* 263–269.

Roden, M. and Simmons, B.B. (2014) 'Delirium superimposed on dementia and mild cognitive impairment.' *Postgraduate Medicine 126,* 6, 129–137. Available at www.ncbi.nlm.nih.gov/pubmed/25414941, accessed on 16 August 2016.

Rogers, J. (2007) 'Design for Learning.' In J. Rogers, *Adults Learning* (5th edn). Maidenhead: Open University Press.

Romero, J.P., Benito-León, J., Louis, E.D. and Bermejo-Pareja, F. (2014) 'Under reporting of dementia deaths on death certificates: A systematic review of population-based cohort studies.' *Journal of Alzheimer's Disease 41,* 1, 213–221.

Rowlands, C. and Rowlands, J. (2012) 'Challenges in delivering effective palliative care to people with dementia.' *Mental Health Practice 16,* 4, 33–36.

Ruddon, R.W. (2010) *Molecular Biology of Cancer: Translation to the Clinic.* Leiden, the Netherlands: Academic Press.

Ruggeri, K., Farrington, C. and Brayne, C. (2013) 'A global model for effective use and evaluation of e-learning in health.' *Telemedicine Journal and e-Health: The Official Journal of the American Telemedicine Association 19,* 4, 312–321.

Russell, S. (2014a) 'Advance care planning: Whose agenda is it anyway?' *Palliative Medicine 28,* 8, 997–999.

Russell, S. (2014b) *Summary of BHL, ABC End of Life Education Programme.* Health Education East of England/Hospice of St Francis.

Russell, S. (2015) 'Do definitions matter in palliative care?' *International Journal of Palliative Nursing 21,* 4, 160–161.

Russell, S. (2016) 'Getting the most out of End of Life Care for All (e-ELCA) e-learning.' Available at www.ehospice.com/uk/Default/tabid/10697/ArticleId/18575, accessed on 22 September 2016.

Ryan, T., Gardiner, C., Bellamy, G., Gott, M. and Ingleton, C. (2012) 'Barriers and facilitators to the receipt of palliative care for people with dementia: The views of medical and nursing staff.' *Palliative Medicine 26,* 879–886.

Sampson, E.L., Gould, V., Lee, D. and Blanchard, M.R. (2006) 'Differences in care received by patients with and without dementia who died during acute hospital admission: A retrospective case note study.' *Age and Ageing 35,* 187–189.

Sampson, E.L., White, N., Lord, K., Leurent, B. *et al.* (2015) 'Pain, agitation, and behavioural problems in people with dementia admitted to general hospital wards: A longitudinal cohort study.' *Pain 156,* 4, 675–683.

Saunders, C. (1967) *The Management of Terminal Illness.* London: Hospital Medicine Publications.

Schön, D.A. (1983) *The Reflective Practitioner: How Professionals Think in Action.* New York: Basic Books.

SCIE (Social Care Institute for Excellence) (2009) 'The Open Dementia Programme: Module 7 – Positive Communication.' Available at www.scie. org.uk/publications/elearning/dementia/dementia07/resource/flash/index.html, accessed on 17 September 2016.

SCIE (2012) 'End of life care in dementia.' Available at www.scie.org.uk/publications/dementia/endoflife/last.asp, accessed on 16 August 2016.

Shanley, C., Russell, C., Middleton, H. and Simpson-Young, V. (2011) 'Living through end-stage dementia: The experiences and expressed needs of family carers.' *Dementia 10,* 3, 325–340.

Shega, J., Levin, A., Hougham, G., Cox-Hayley, D. *et al.* (2003) 'Palliative Excellence in Alzheimer Care Efforts (PEACE): A program description.' *Journal of Palliative Medicine 6,* 315–320.

Shershneva, M.B., Wang, M.F., Lindeman, G.C., Savoy, J.N. and Olson, C.A. (2010) 'Commitment to practice change: An evaluator's perspective.' *Evaluation and the Health Professions 33,* 3, 256–275.

Shotton, L. and Seedhouse, D. (1998) 'Practical dignity in caring.' *Nursing Ethics 5,* 246–255.

Skills for Care and Skills for Health (2014) *Common Core Principles and Competences for Social Care and Health Workers Working with Adults at the End of Life* (2nd edition). Leeds: Skills for Care and Skills for Health. Available at www.skillsforcare.org.uk/Documents/Topics/End-of-life-care/Common-core-principles-and-competences-for-social-care-and-health-workers-working-with-adults-at-the-end-of-life.pdf, accessed on 22 September 2016.

Skills for Care and Skills for Health and DH (2011) 'Common core principles for supporting people with dementia: A guide to training the social care and health workforce.' Available at www.skillsforcare.org.uk/Document-library/Skills/Dementia/CCP-Dementia-(webv2)%5B1%5D.pdf, accessed on 22 September 2016.

Slatten, L.A., Carson, K.D. and Carson, P.P. (2011) 'Compassion fatigue and burnout: What managers should know.' *The Health Care Manager 30,* 4, 325–333.

Smale, B. and Dupuis, S.L. (2004) *Caregivers of Persons with Dementia: Roles, Experiences, Supports and Coping.* A literature review.

Snow, A.L., O'Malley, K.J., Cody, M., Kunik, M.E. *et al.* (2004) 'A conceptual model of pain assessment for noncommunicative persons with dementia.' *The Gerontologist 44,* 6, 807–817.

Sommerbakk, R., Haugen, D.F., Tjora, A., Kaasa, S. and Hjermstad, M.J. (2016) 'Barriers to and facilitators for implementing quality improvements in palliative care – Results from a qualitative interview study in Norway.' *BMC Palliative Care 15,* 1, 61.

Spilsbury, K., Hanratty, B. and McCaughan, D. (2015) *Supporting Nursing in Care Homes*. Project Report for the RCN Foundation. University of York.

Stedeford, A. (1987) 'Hospice: A safe place to suffer?' *Palliative Medicine 1*, 1, 73–74.

Stroebe, M.S., Stroebe, W. and Hansson, R.O. (1993) *Handbook of Bereavement: Theory, Research, and Intervention*. New York: Cambridge University Press.

Summersall, J. and Wight, S. (2004) 'When it's difficult to swallow: The role of the speech therapist.' *Nursing and Residential Care 6*, 11, 550–553.

Sykes, J.B. (1979) *The Concise Oxford Dictionary of Current English*. London: Book Club Associates.

Teno, J.M., Weitzen, S., Fennell, M.L. and Mor, V. (2001) 'Dying trajectory in the last year of life: Does cancer trajectory fit other diseases?' *Journal of Palliative Medicine 4*, 4, 457–464.

The Choice in End of Life Care Programme Board (2015) 'What's important to me: A review of choice in end of life care.' Available at www.gov.uk/government/uploads/system/uploads/attachment_data/file/407244/CHOICE_REVIEW_FINAL_for_web.pdf, accessed on 22 September 2016.

Thomas, K. (2010) 'Using prognostic indicator guidance to plan care for the final stages of life.' *Primary Health Care 20*, 25–28.

Thompson, R. and Heath, H. (2013) *Dementia: Commitment to the Care of People with Dementia in Hospital Settings*. London: Royal College of Nursing.

Titchen, A., Dewing, J. and Manley, K. (2013) 'Getting Going with Facilitation Skills in Practice Development.' In B. McCormack, K. Manley and A. Titchen (eds) *Practice Development in Nursing and Healthcare* (2nd edn). Oxford: Wiley-Blackwell.

Tolman, S. (2015) 'Admiral nursing in a hospice.' Available at www.ehospice.com/uk/Default/tabid/10697/ArticleId/14477, accessed on 16 August 2016.

Toot, S., Devine, M., Akporobaro, A. and Orrell, M. (2013) 'Causes of hospital admission for people with dementia: A systematic review and meta-analysis.' *Journal of the American Medical Directors Association 14*, 7, 463–470.

Travis, S.S., Conway, J., Daly, M. and Larsen, P. (2001) 'Terminal restlessness in the nursing facility: Assessment, palliation, and symptom management.' *Geriatric Nursing 22*, 6, 308–312.

Treloar, A., Crugel, M. and Adamis, D. (2009) 'Palliative and end of life care of dementia at home is feasible and rewarding: Results from the "Hope for Home" study.' *Dementia 8*, 335–347. Available at http://dem.sagepub.com/content/8/3/335.short, accessed on 9 August 2016.

Treloar, A., Crugel, M., Prasanna, A., Solomons, L. *et al.* (2010) 'Ethical dilemmas: Should antipsychotics ever be prescribed for people with dementia?' *The British Journal of Psychiatry 197*, 2, 88–90.

Twycross, R. and Wilcock, A. (2001) 'Pain Relief.' In R. Twycross and A. Wilcock, *Symptom Management in Advanced Cancer* (3rd edn). Oxon: Radcliffe Medical Press.

van der Steen, J.T. (2010) 'Dying with dementia: What we know after more than a decade of research.' *Journal of Alzheimer's Disease 22*, 1, 37–55.

van der Steen, J.T., Radbruch, L., Hertogh, C.M., de Boer, M.E. *et al.* (2013) 'White paper defining optimal palliative care in older people with dementia: A Delphi study and recommendations from the European Association for Palliative Care.' *Palliative Medicine 28*, 3, 197–209.

Volicer, L. and Hurley, A. (2004) *Hospice Care for Patients with Advanced Progressive Dementia.* New York: Springer Publishing Company.

Walsh, K. (2011) *Grief and Loss: Theories and Skills for the Helping Professions.* London: Pearson.

Watson, J., Hockley, J. and Murray, S. (2010) 'Evaluating effectiveness of the GSFCH and LCP in care homes.' *End of Life Care Journal 4*, 3, 42–49.

Wee, B. (2012) 'Can e-learning be used to teach end-of-life care?' *BMJ Supportive and Palliative Care 2*, 4, 292–293.

WHO (World Health Organization) (1998) 'WHO definition of palliative care.' Available at www.who.int/cancer/palliative/definition/en, accessed on 16 August 2016.

Wilden, B.M. and Wright, N.E. (2002) 'Concept of pre-death restlessness in dementia.' *Journal of Gerontological Nursing 28*, 10, 24–29.

Wilson, J., O'Donnell, M., McAuliffe, L., Nay, R. and Pitcher, A. (2008) *Assessment of Pain in Older Adults with Dementia in Acute, Sub Acute and Residential Care (Systematic Review).* Australian Centre for Evidence Based Aged Care, La Trobe University.

Worden, J.W. (1992) *Grief Counselling and Grief Therapy: A Handbook for the Mental Health Practitioner* (2nd edn). London: Tavistock/Routledge.

Zarit, S.H. and Zarit, J.M. (2008) 'Flexibility and Change: The Fundamentals for Families Coping with Dementia.' In M. Downs and B. Bowers (eds) *Excellence in Dementia Care: Research into Practice.* Maidenhead: Open University Press.

# Subject Index

# Author Index